Sideline Help

Marshall K. Steele III, MD
President, Orthopaedic and Sports Medicine Center
Annapolis, MD

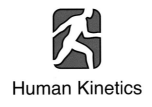

Human Kinetics

Library of Congress Cataloging-in-Publication Data

Steele, Marshall K., 1946-
    Sideline help / Marshall K. Steele.
        p.   cm.
    ISBN 0-87322-786-7
    1. Sports injuries.   2. First aid in illness and injury.
    I. Title.
    RD97.S84   1996
    617.1'027--dc20   95-38863
                                                                        CIP

ISBN: 0-87322-786-7

Copyright © 1996 by Marshall K. Steele III

Developmental Editor: Larret Galasyn-Wright
Managing Editor: Julie Marx Ohnemus
Copyeditor: Holly Gilly
Proofreader: Jim Burns
Designer and Illustrator: Doug Burnett
Typesetter and Layout Artist: Kathy Boudreau-Fuoss
Silhouette Illustrator: Keith Blomberg
Cover Designer: Jack Davis
Cover Photographer: ©Wilmer Zehr

Human Kinetics books are available at special discounts for bulk purchase. Special editions or book excerpts can also be created to specification. For details, contact the Special Sales Manager at Human Kinetics.

Printed in Hong Kong

10 9 8 7 6 5 4 3 2 1

Human Kinetics
P.O. Box 5076, Champaign, IL 61825-5076
1-800-747-4457

Canada: Human Kinetics, Box 24040, Windsor, ON N8Y 4Y9
1-800-465-7301 (in Canada only)

Europe: Human Kinetics, P.O. Box IW14, Leeds LS16 6TR, United Kingdom
(44) 1132 781708

Australia: Human Kinetics, 2 Ingrid Street, Clapham 5062, South Australia
(08) 371 3755

New Zealand: Human Kinetics, P.O. Box 105-231, Auckland 1
(09) 523 3462

To my father, Marshall Steele Jr., MD,
who inspired my interest in sports and medicine,
and to my mother, Elsie Steele,
who taught me to finish what I started.

Contents

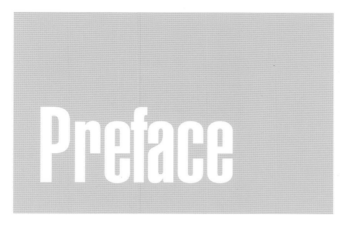

Preface

This year the U.S. Consumer Product Safety Commission estimates that hospital emergency rooms will treat four million young athletes for sports-related injuries and that eight million more injuries from the playing fields will be treated by family physicians. For those of us watching or coaching young athletes from the sidelines, these are staggering statistics. In the event of an injury, are you equipped to help? Most youth coaches and parents are not.

For the young athletes under your supervision, and for you, the first 10 minutes following an injury are critical. Whether at home, on the playground, or on the court or field, if a medical professional is unavailable, *you* must take charge of the situation. The decisions you make and the actions you take are vital to the well-being of an injured athlete. Therefore, you must be prepared, even for a life-threatening injury.

This book will help you make the right decisions in an injury situation.

In *Sideline Help* I cover all the common sports injuries, ranging from minor ankle sprains to serious head injuries. For each injury I've created an easy-to-use, color-coded flowchart that guides you through a five-step on-field and sideline evaluation process. This process is designed to help you determine

  the type of injury sustained,

  the athlete's physical and mental status,

  the severity of the injury,

    whether or not to call for emergency help,

    whether or not the athlete should be taken to a doctor,

    what, if any, first aid procedures should be started, and

    whether or not it is safe for the athlete to return to play.

This process is not a substitute for professional medical assistance. Instead, it is designed to help you determine if you need to call for experienced medical personnel and to assist you in caring for an injured athlete until such help arrives. Always defer to medical personnel if they are present.

As a parent, physician, and sports enthusiast who for the last 20 years has spent countless hours on the sidelines at athletic events, I came to believe that a simple, easy-to-use sports injury manual for nonphysicians was desperately needed. I wrote *Sideline Help* for you, the coaches, teachers, and parents who each season are responsible for supervising young athletes at practice and play. It is my sincerest hope that you will find this book informative and useful both on the field and off and that it will help you better care for injured athletes during those first 10 minutes when they need you most.

Acknowledgments

I appreciate the many people who helped and encouraged me in the writing of this book. I am indebted to Robert Kramer and Amy Dembinsky of Kramer & Associates, to my developmental editor Larret Galasyn-Wright at Human Kinetics, to Marti Betz for her help in the early stages of the project, and to my wife, Susan. Without their help this guide would never have been completed.

I would also like to thank Tom Harries, MD, who encouraged me to persevere, as well as the other coaches and friends who supported my endeavor, including Greg Hrebiniak, Ken Dunn, Pat Bryan, Sue Patton, Annie Kramer, Chuck Dillman, Sim Wooten, Skip Weitzen, Bill and Kathy Simms, and my children, John, Julianne, and David Steele.

In addition, I appreciate the efforts of sports trainers Rob Patterson, Sue Payne, and Melinda Flegel and physicians Dan McCabe, Bob Noel, Ray Herzinger, Steve Hiltabidle, Tom Ducker, and Karl Holschuh in reviewing the manuscript and giving me feedback.

Finally, I owe special thanks to the Anne Arundel County coaches, especially to Paul Rusko and Mike Busch, who work to help make our sports programs safer.

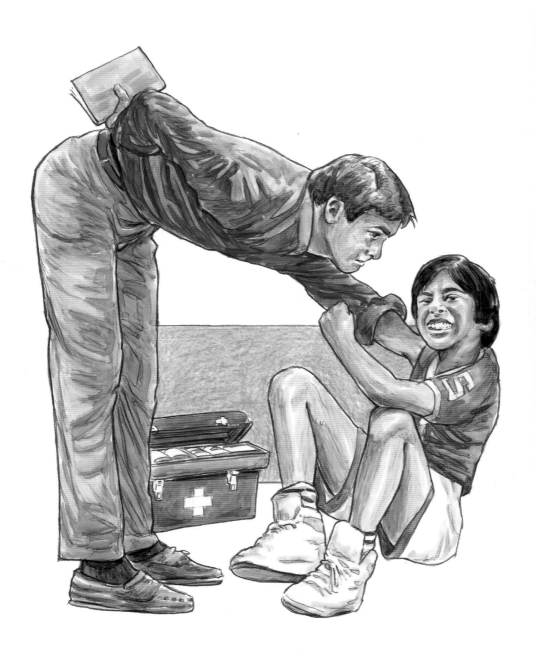

How to Use This Book

This book is designed to be a *quick* reference to help you in your evaluation of an injured athlete. In order to use this guide as it is intended, it is essential that you familiarize yourself with the content of *Sideline Help* so you are able to quickly locate information about specific injuries. You also need to develop the skills necessary to follow the emergency guidelines that are provided. As you use the preseason months to plan new workouts and strategies, be sure to allow time to prepare yourself with the knowledge and skills you will need in an emergency situation. It is very important to become certified in both cardiopulmonary resuscitation (CPR) and first aid—whether or not you possess the skills taught in these courses can mean the difference between life and death for an injured athlete in your care. Contact any of the organizations listed at the end of this book for assistance if you have difficulty locating an injury prevention workshop or a CPR or first aid course in your area.

After you become familiar with the structure of *Sideline Help*, the order in which material is presented, and the decisions you will make while following the flowcharts for each injury, your next goal should be to learn what steps to take before each game to ensure efficient emergency procedures. The following sections contain information to help you accomplish these goals.

Before the Game

There are several steps you should take before every game to help you handle any emergency situation effectively. By taking the time to address the following issues before an injury occurs, you can be confident that procedures are in place to help carry out your decisions quickly and efficiently. Then, if an emergency does occur, you will be able to concentrate your full attention on helping the injured athlete.

▓ Identify any trained medical personnel in attendance.

▓ If you are not certified in CPR, make sure someone at the game is.

▓ Designate an assistant to help you in case of an emergency. (Ideally, this should be someone who is able to help you throughout the season and who is as familiar with CPR, first aid, and the procedures listed in *Sideline Help* as you are.)

▓ Study the playing area and determine how an emergency vehicle could access the field or building.

▓ Locate the nearest telephone or arrange to have a cellular phone available.

▓ Check and restock your first aid kit. Take your first aid kit to every game and practice; a well-stocked kit could mean the difference between an athlete's receiving effective treatment or sustaining permanent injury. Every kit should contain the following items, which should be stored in a well-organized, easily accessible carrying case.

  ▓ Adhesive bandages (assorted sizes)
  ▓ Bleach and water solution made up of 1 part household bleach to 10 parts water
  ▓ Cardboard splints, pillows, or a commercial splint
  ▓ Elastic wraps (2, 4, and 6 inches wide)
  ▓ Finger splints
  ▓ Gauze pads
  ▓ Hydrogen peroxide to clean wounds
  ▓ Instant ice packs

- Isopropyl alcohol to clean wounds
- Latex gloves
- List of athletes with special conditions
- List of emergency medical service numbers if 911 service is not available
- List of your athletes' emergency contact numbers
- Penlight
- Scissors
- *Sideline Help*
- Sling
- Triple antibiotic ointment
- White athletic tape (1 and 2 inches wide)
- Wound-care spray to sterilize wounds

Sideline Help at a Glance

I've divided *Sideline Help* into two sections. The first section, "Basic Knowledge and Essential Skills," should serve as a review of the skills you need to learn in the care and prevention workshops that you attend before the season begins. The second section—the section you will use the most when evaluating injured athletes— consists of flowcharts that guide you through the evaluation and care process for all of the most common sports injuries. The injury section is divided into four parts—Critical Injuries, Internal Organ Injuries, Facial Injuries, and Extremity Injuries—each of which is marked with a different color along the side and top of the book for easy reference. Each part begins with general information to keep in mind as you evaluate for any of the injuries in that part; in turn, each injury flowchart begins with information dealing specifically with that injury, including unique signs or symptoms to look for, possible injuries you might find, and several of "Dr. Steele's Quick Tips" to help you with your evaluation. Familiarize yourself with these introductory sections for each part and injury before the season begins, even before every game if necessary—chances are you won't have time to refer to them during an emergency.

    Sideline Help will guide you through the process of determining the seriousness of the injury the athlete has received and help you decide how to proceed once you have made that determination. The flowchart for each injury will guide you step-by-step through this process from your initial contact with the injured athlete on the field to your final decision of whether or not the athlete can return to play. Since your initial evaluation will be completed on the playing area and the follow-up evaluation will take place after the athlete has been removed from the game, each injury flowchart is divided into two parts: on-field evaluation and sideline evaluation. Always start your evaluation with the on-field flowchart, and never return an athlete to play without further evaluation on the sideline. Throughout the process, remember that this guide is not intended to replace professional medical care, and if at any point in your evaluation the help of experienced professionals becomes available, defer to their judgment.

As you read through *Sideline Help*, you will see that the decisions you must make and the questions you must ask yourself when evaluating each injury are the same. If you are evaluating an athlete on-field, is the injury serious enough to call for emergency help or can the athlete be moved to the sideline? Once the athlete is safely on the sideline and you begin further evaluation, are there any signs or symptoms that require emergency care? Are there less serious indications of injury that will require the athlete to see a doctor? Has the athlete recovered, and does she want to return to play? Is the potential seriousness of the injury so great that, even if the athlete appears to be unharmed, return to play is not an option? The checklists within each injury flowchart will guide you through this decision-making process by providing you with signs and symptoms to look for, specific emergency care guidelines to follow, steps to take when moving the athlete off the field, and the criteria each athlete must meet before the decision to return to play can be made.

Remember, the first 10 minutes after an injury are critical, and your quick, correct response is essential. To help your athletes when they need you the most, you need to be able to handle emergencies effectively and confidently. And with the proper courses in first aid and CPR, and with *Sideline Help* as your guide, you *can* make the decisions necessary to save a life and avoid further injury!

Basic Knowledge and Essential Skills

Do you know how to check mental status after an injury, how to properly assist the athlete from the field, and how to handle blood safely? You need to know the answers to these and other questions in order to follow the guidelines for treating injuries in Parts 1 through 4 of this handbook. These skills are best learned by attending a hands-on care and prevention workshop in your area. This section of the manual is designed to reinforce the skills you have learned in such a workshop.

Eight Important Checks

For each injury you will be prompted to evaluate the athlete for certain signs and symptoms. *Signs* are findings you observe in the athlete by looking or examining, such as unconsciousness or lack of a pulse. *Symptoms* are answers to the questions you ask the athlete or information the athlete volunteers. For example, pain and nausea are symptoms. Eight important checks you should include in the evaluation of any injured athlete are explained in the next few pages.

Checking for Mental Status

You must be able to assess the mental status of an athlete. Head injury, heat stroke, blood loss, shock, and low blood sugar are some of the most common injuries and conditions that can alter mental status. Altered mental status is an important sign of injury, and you must carefully assess even the most minor change. Take your time and be thorough when you check for the following:

- *Lack of alertness.* Unconsciousness or lack of alertness may be a sign of serious brain dysfunction.

- *Agitation.* Belligerence or uncooperative behavior may also be a sign of disturbed brain function. This may manifest itself when the athlete

  - acts combative and angry,
  - wants to get up when you ask her to be still, or
  - uses foul language.

- *Incorrect response.* Checking the athlete's ability to process information and perform motor skills is a way for you to evaluate mental status and nerve function at the same time. Use the four-extremity test to check for dysfunction. Ask the athlete to

  - grip with the right hand, then lift the right arm,
  - grip with the left hand, then lift the left arm,
  - wiggle the right foot, then lift the right leg, and
  - wiggle the left foot, then lift the left leg.

Do not ask the athlete to lift an arm or leg if there is evidence of serious arm or leg injury.

- *Memory loss.* Recent memory loss is a subtle but important sign in assessing brain function. Ask the athlete these questions:
  - "How did this injury occur?"
  - "Where are you?"
  - "What is the score [or time]?"
  - "Who are you playing?"

Checking for Shock

Check for shock with any serious injury. Shock is a medical term that describes a lowering of the blood pressure to dangerous levels, and it should be treated as a medical emergency. Cardiac dysfunction, blood loss, heat stroke, and serious head or neck injury can all lead to shock. In addition, severe pain sometimes causes a reaction in the body that can lead to fainting and shock. There are several signs and symptoms of shock:

- Pulse greater than 120 beats per minute
- Profuse sweating
- Cool, clammy skin
- Dizziness
- Paleness
- Nausea or vomiting

Checking for Pulse

Why is the pulse important? An absent neck pulse indicates that the heart has stopped and emergency procedures must begin. In extremity injuries, a strong pulse at the wrist or ankle will tell you that blood is flowing freely to the extremity, and an absent pulse may indicate a blood vessel has been compressed or ruptured. A weak pulse or pulse greater than 120 beats per minute may indicate shock with rapid internal or external blood loss.

Using a watch for timing accuracy, take the athlete's pulse at the neck, wrist, or ankle for 15 seconds and multiply by four to estimate the beats per minute. If you have trouble feeling a pulse, take the pulse at another site to compare.

I recommend you take a pulse at the following sites for these injuries:

- For an unconscious athlete, check the pulse at the neck.

- For an upper extremity injury, check the pulse at the wrist.

- For a lower extremity injury, check the pulse at the back of the ankle just behind the inside bone or at the top of the ankle.

Checking for Numbness

If you see no obvious serious injury, test for numbness by touching the athlete lightly with the tip of your finger or a pen. **Do not test for numbness if you have already observed a serious injury. Instead, follow the Emergency Care Guidelines to avoid further damage.**

Spinal and extremity injuries may injure nerves, which will cause both numbness and weakness. Consider athletes who report tingling in their arms or legs to have a nerve or spinal injury. For suspected neck injuries you must test both hands and feet. In extremity injuries, compare limbs to evaluate the degree of numbness in the injured one using the following procedures. However, in head and spinal injuries this comparison will not be helpful because both limbs may be affected.

Lower Extremity

- First, touch the big toe and ask the athlete to identify which toe you are touching.

- As you touch the remaining toes, ask the athlete to rate the sensation on a scale of 1 to 10 and to identify which toe you are touching.

- Touch the front of the ankle and move upward to touch the front and back of the lower leg.

- Touch the front and then the back of the thigh.

Upper Extremity

▪ Start with the thumb and ask the athlete to identify which finger you are touching.

▪ As you touch each finger, ask the athlete to rate the sensation on a scale of 1 to 10 and to identify which finger you are touching.

▪ As you touch the front and back of the forearm, then the upper arm, and finally the top of the shoulder, ask the athlete to rate the sensation on a scale of 1 to 10.

Checking for Strength

If you see no obvious serious injury, evaluate for strength. **Do not test for strength if you have already observed a serious injury. Instead, follow the Emergency Care Guidelines to avoid further damage.**

Spinal or extremity injuries may compress or lacerate nerves. Such nerve injuries can be detected by noting weakness or paralysis of muscles supplied by the nerves. Muscle weakness may also be caused by pain, direct injury to the muscle itself, or rupture of an associated tendon. Do not allow any athlete who hasn't regained normal strength to return to play. Evaluate strength in the injured limb by comparing it with the opposite limb. Test muscles for strength by following these procedures.

Shoulder

▪ Have the athlete lift the elbow out to the side at shoulder height. Push down against the elbow while the athlete resists.

▪ Have the athlete hold the elbow against his side with the forearm straight forward. Push the athlete's hand outward then inward while he resists.

Elbow

▪ Have the athlete straighten the elbow and then bend it while you provide resistance.

▪ Have the athlete bend the elbow 90 degrees and then straighten it while you provide resistance.

Wrist

- Have the athlete pull the wrist back. Try to bend the athlete's wrist down while asking her to resist you.

- Have the athlete bend the wrist down. Have the athlete bend the wrist back up while you provide resistance.

Hand

- Have the athlete straighten the fingers.

- Have the athlete grip tightly.

Hip

- Have the athlete lie on his back, lift the leg off the ground, and hold it there while you try to push it back down.

- Have the athlete walk to see if there is limping.

Knee

- Have the athlete straighten the knee. Try to bend the athlete's knee while asking him to hold it straight.

- Have the athlete bend the knee 90 degrees. Try to straighten the athlete's knee while asking him to keep it bent.

Ankle/Foot

- Have the athlete pull the foot and toes up. Try to pull the athlete's foot and toes down while she resists.

- Have the athlete push the foot and toes down. Try to push the athlete's foot and toes up while she resists.

Checking for Localized Tenderness

If you see no obvious serious injury, test for localized or point tenderness. **Do not test for localized tenderness if you have already observed a serious injury. Instead, follow the Emergency Care Guidelines to avoid further damage.**

Localized tenderness precisely identifies the injured area, and it is often a sign of a fracture. Push gently around the injured area with your index finger or thumb. Ask the athlete to grade the pain from 1 to 10. When you find an area that grades high (8 to 10), note that area. Then touch gently in an area 1 to 2 inches around this tender area. An athlete has localized tenderness when the surrounding area rates low (1-5) and the tender area rates high (8-10).

Checking for Range of Motion

If there is no obvious serious injury, test for painful or limited range of motion. **Do not test the range of motion if you have already observed a serious injury. Instead, follow the Emergency Care Guidelines to avoid further damage.**

Loss of motion or pain with motion indicates a potentially significant injury to the joint or structures near the joint. Compare opposite limbs to evaluate if range of motion is limited in the injured one. Ask the athlete to slowly move the suspected injured joint in the ways described below.

Neck

- Touch the chin to the right shoulder.
- Touch the chin to the left shoulder.
- Touch the chin to the chest.
- Tilt the head back.

Back

- Touch the toes.
- Bend to the right, then left.
- Lean back.

Shoulder

- Raise the arm completely to the side and touch the opposite ear.
- Reach up behind the back.

Elbow

- Fully straighten the elbow and turn the palm up, then down.
- Bend the elbow up completely to touch the shoulder with the hand.

Wrist

▪ Pull the wrist completely back and bend it completely down.

▪ Turn the palm up and down.

Fingers

▪ Straighten the fingers and thumb fully.

▪ Completely bend the fingers and thumb so that the tips touch the crease in the palm.

Hip

▪ Bend the knee fully into the chest.

▪ Straighten the leg completely.

▪ Rotate the hip by rolling the leg in and out.

Knee

▪ Straighten the knee fully.

▪ Bend the knee fully.

Ankle/Foot

▪ Pull the foot and toes up fully.

▪ Push the foot and toes down fully.

▪ Move the foot from side to side.

Checking for Grating Bones

If there is no obvious serious injury, test for grating. **Do not test for grating if you have already observed a serious injury. Instead, follow the Emergency Care Guidelines to avoid further damage.**

When a bone breaks or dislocates (goes out of joint), the two ends may rub together and grate or crunch. Put your hand over the injured area and ask the athlete to move the joint. If you feel a grating, grinding, or crunching, a fracture or dislocation is likely. If you do not feel grating, gently grasp above and below the injured area with both hands and carefully move the bone to feel for grating. Do not feel for grating if there is significant pain at rest or during movement; proceed immediately to the Emergency Care Guidelines in this case.

Emergency Care Guidelines

Call 911 if an injury is serious and requires immediate, professional medical attention. Limit further evaluation to determining the need for cardiopulmonary resuscitation (CPR), treatment for shock, controlling severe bleeding, and immobilizing the athlete. Evaluation beyond these determinations could cause more harm and delay. Your goal while waiting for help is to preserve life and limb and to protect the athlete from further injury.

Calling 911

When confronted with a downed athlete on the field, your first decision is whether or not you should call 911. Calling 911 has three basic purposes: preserving life and limb, preventing further injury, and ensuring a safe and comfortable transfer to a medical care facility. This decision is best made by the medical personnel at the game. However, if no one is available, the decision may be yours alone. Do not delay calling 911 when there is reason.

Dr. Steele's Quick Tips

- If you are unsure about calling 911, make the call.
- Time is of the essence in preserving life and limb and preventing further injury. Call 911 immediately if the athlete shows any of these signs:
  - Unconsciousness or altered mental status
  - Problems with breathing
  - Possible cardiac arrest
  - Shock
  - Severe bleeding
  - Possible head, neck, or back injury
  - Possible heat stroke
  - Possible internal organ injury

- No pulse in an injured extremity
- Numbness of an extremity

- Ensuring a safe transfer while preventing further injury is especially important with extremity injuries. Always call 911 when the athlete has these conditions:

  - Severe pain
  - Deformity
  - Open or puncture wound near a suspected fracture
  - Cannot be assisted from the field

- With some injuries, you may need to choose between calling 911 and transporting the athlete to a medical facility yourself. These injuries include the following:

  - Eye injuries
  - Nose injuries
  - Jaw injuries
  - Extremity injuries showing signs of weakness, localized tenderness, painful range of motion, or grating bones

Every medical situation is different. Whether you choose to call 911 or to transport the athlete to a medical facility yourself will depend on the seriousness of each injury, your level of medical training, skills you have mastered, and your experience with injuries.

Cardiopulmonary Arrest

When an athlete is unconscious, have someone call 911 while you evaluate for cardiac or pulmonary arrest. Cardiac arrest occurs when the heart has stopped beating. In this situation, the athlete quickly becomes unconscious and breathing stops or becomes irregular. Pulmonary arrest occurs when breathing stops. If the heartbeat and breathing stop for more than four to six minutes, permanent damage or death may occur. The American Heart Association teaches the *ABC* method of evaluation and cardiopulmonary resuscitation (CPR). You must become certified in both to be able to evaluate and treat athletes with cardiac or pulmonary problems. If you are not certified, quickly find someone who is and let her assume responsibility. The *ABC*s stand for **a**irway, **b**reathing, and **C**irculation.

■ **A**irway. Is the airway clear so that the athlete can breathe? Is breathing obstructed and noisy?

■ **B**reathing. Is the athlete breathing? Look closely for movement of the chest and abdomen. Feel for air coming out of the nose and mouth.

■ **C**irculation. Is there a pulse at the neck or wrist? Once cardiac arrest occurs or breathing stops, you have only four to six minutes to initiate CPR. This is why it is so essential for you to be certified.

Dr. Steele's Quick Tips

■ Get certified in CPR. It could save a life.

Treating for Shock

Shock occurs when blood pressure drops to dangerous levels. This causes rapid pulse, profuse sweating, cool and clammy skin, dizziness, paleness, nausea, and vomiting. Treating for shock includes identifying and treating its underlying cause and reducing its effects on the body.

There are multiple causes for shock, including cardiac dysfunction, blood loss, heat stroke, and head or neck injury. Severe pain or fear can also cause a shock-like reaction that produces fainting.

You can reduce the effects of shock on the body by getting more blood to the heart and brain. This is best accomplished in two ways:

■ Laying the athlete down flat and elevating the legs three to six inches to allow the blood to flow toward the heart

■ Keeping the athlete comfortably warm

If you suspect a spinal injury, do not move the athlete. In cases of heat stroke, don't warm the athlete further. Instead, douse her with cold water and fan her with towels to cool her down.

No Food or Water

Any athlete who is injured and is being sent to the hospital may require surgery. Anesthesia cannot be administered safely if the athlete has liquid or solid food in his stomach. Therefore, refrain from giving the seriously injured athlete anything to eat or drink unless you are treating heat exhaustion, heat stroke, or hypoglycemia. Hypoglycemia (low blood sugar) occasionally occurs in people with diabetes who require insulin. If you have an athlete with diabetes, communicate with the athlete's parents and doctor so you will recognize the signs of hypoglycemia. Have a sugared drink available for these athletes.

Bleeding Injuries

When dealing with open wounds and bleeding, you must consider these three things:

- Stopping the bleeding and protecting the wound from contamination
- Protecting yourself from contamination
- Protecting others from contamination

Minor wounds are very common and you must know the proper steps to handling the bleeding associated with them.

Dr. Steele's Quick Tips

- Do not probe a wound, because this will increase the bleeding.

Guidelines for Handling Blood*

Blood may carry with it viruses such as hepatitis and AIDS that can be transmitted when blood from one athlete comes into contact with an open cut on another person. Small cuts can occur on the arms and

*Adapted from American Medical Society for Sports Medicine and the American Academy of Sports Medicine, 1995, "Human immunodeficiency virus and other blood-borne pathogens in sports," *Clinical Journal of Sports Medicine* **5**(3): 202-203.

legs of athletes without being noticed. Therefore, everyone is at risk when an athlete sustains a cut that bleeds.

Any risk of blood-borne disease transmission in sport is exceedingly small. However, anyone involved with sport will help further reduce the risk of transmission by following guidelines that are both practical and simple to implement. A major component of these guidelines is common sense and adherence to basic principles of hygiene.

Because the risk of blood-borne disease transmission in sport is confined to contact with blood, body fluids, and other fluids containing blood, focus on recognizing and treating bleeding immediately using the following guidelines.

- Cover abrasions, cuts, or oozing wounds with an absorbing dressing.

- Remove participants with active bleeding from the event as soon as possible. When bleeding is controlled and the wound is properly covered, the player may return to competition, but if the uniform is saturated with blood, the athlete must change it before returning to competition.

- Wear latex or vinyl gloves when you anticipate direct contact with blood, body fluids, and other fluids containing blood.

- Clean and cover minor cuts and abrasions that are not bleeding during scheduled breaks in play.

- Wipe immediately with paper towels or disposable cloths any equipment or area soiled with blood. Disinfect the contaminated areas with a solution prepared with 1 part household bleach to 10 parts water. Prepare a fresh solution daily.

Caring for Major Wounds

A fracture that punctures the skin is called an *open*, or *compound*, *fracture*. This type of fracture or a deep laceration may cause injury to arteries or veins. Arterial bleeding is bright red, bleeds fast, and may pulsate with the beating of the heart. This bleeding is very serious and may threaten the life of the injured athlete. Stop this bleeding by applying pressure directly over where you see the most rapid bleeding. Venous bleeding is dark red and bleeds slowly. This bleeding should also be stopped with direct pressure over the bleeding area. Put on latex gloves, then apply the pressure with sterile gauze sponges. Press hard for about 10 minutes without releasing the pressure to allow a clot to form. When bleeding stops, wrap an elastic bandage around the sponges to hold them in place. If the sponges soak through with blood, do not remove them, because you may disturb the clot that is forming. Instead, add more sponges on top of the blood-soaked ones and press harder until bleeding stops. If bleeding continues to be rapid and uncontrolled, and you believe the athlete is bleeding to death, you may apply a tourniquet as a last resort. Applying a tourniquet improperly may cause further damage to the extremity. Proper tourniquet application is a hands-on skill that must be learned in an appropriate course.

Dr. Steele's Quick Tips

- Call 911 in cases of severe bleeding.

- Wear latex gloves.

- Place gauze sponges over the wound and apply firm pressure for at least 10 minutes.

- Do not remove blood-soaked sponges, but add more and apply firmer pressure.

- If bleeding stops, apply an elastic bandage around the gauze sponges to hold them in place.

- Do not remove gauze sponges.

- If bleeding cannot be stopped and is life threatening, apply a tourniquet as a last resort, if you've been trained.

Splinting

If an extremity injury is serious and the athlete is on the field, avoid moving the injured extremity, call 911, and wait for help. Defer to trained medical personnel to splint the extremity before moving the athlete; do not attempt to splint it yourself. In less serious extremity injuries or when the athlete is on the sideline, splinting the injury will reduce pain and prevent further injury. Splinting is always a two- or three-person job.

Dr. Steele's Quick Tips

■ Have an assistant hold and keep the extremity from moving while you splint.

■ Never wrap an elastic bandage tightly when splinting.

Shoulder/Upper Arm

■ Keep the arm to the side.

■ Place the arm in a sling while keeping the shoulder and arm as still as possible.

■ Wrap an elastic bandage around the arm and body.

Elbow

If the elbow is fairly straight, keep it still.

■ Place a pillow or a cardboard splint from the upper arm to the wrist.

■ Wrap the elbow with an elastic bandage.

If the elbow is bent, keep it still.

■ Place a sling on the arm.

■ Wrap an elastic bandage around the sling and body to hold the elbow still.

Forearm

■ Place a pillow or a piece of cardboard from the elbow to the hand.

■ Wrap the arm with an elastic bandage.

■ Place the arm in a sling.

Hand/Fingers

If there is no serious deformity,

- wrap the injury with an elastic bandage, or
- tape the fingers together, one on each side of the injured finger, unless it is deformed.

If the finger is deformed,

- do not attempt to straighten the deformity, and
- wrap the entire hand gently in an elastic bandage.

Hip/Thigh

- Do not attempt to splint.
- Keep the hip and leg immobile.

Knee/Lower Leg

- Place a pillow, piece of cardboard, or commercial splint from the upper thigh to the ankle.
- Wrap the leg with an elastic bandage.

Ankle/Foot

- Place a pillow, piece of cardboard, or commercial splint behind the leg, from the toes to the knee.
- Wrap the ankle with an elastic bandage.

Assisting an Injured Athlete off the Field

Assist an injured athlete to the sideline only after you have evaluated the athlete carefully on the field and decided that no emergency exists. When the athlete cannot get himself off the field without being carried, wait for trained medical personnel. Assisting the athlete from the field properly ensures that no further injury occurs. Extremity injuries may require splinting before the athlete can be moved.

A lower extremity injury requires a two-person assist, one on each side. Place one of the athlete's arms around the neck of one helper, place the other arm around the neck of the other helper, and support the athlete as she walks off. To transport a player with an upper extremity injury, support his forearm or upper arm against his body and walk with him. Wrap an elastic bandage around the athlete's arm and body to reduce arm movement.

Dr. Steele's Quick Tips

- Only trained medical personnel should carry a seriously injured athlete off the field.

PRICE Guidelines

When the athlete is safely on the sideline and you suspect she has received a soft-tissue injury, such as a severe bruise or a sprained ankle or wrist, or a possible bone fracture, take the following steps, identified by the acronym PRICE:

- **P**rotection. Splint the injury.
- **R**est. Keep the athlete off the injured part.
- **I**ce. Wrap ice in a towel and apply it to swelling for 10 to 15 minutes.
- **C**ompression. Wrap the injured area with elastic bandages.
- **E**levation. Raise the injured extremity above the heart.

Dr. Steele's Quick Tips

- Never use heat immediately after an injury, and never leave ice on an extremity for more than 20 minutes each hour.

Common Minor Injuries

Although minor injuries such as missing or cracked teeth, leg cramps, or getting the wind knocked out don't threaten life or limb, they are still painful for the athlete and they require care.

Missing or Cracked Teeth

A hard blow to the mouth may crack a tooth or knock it completely out, requiring a prompt visit to the dentist. It is possible to save a tooth that is promptly reimplanted. Use the athlete's saliva to moisten a gauze sponge and wrap the tooth in the sponge.

Dr. Steele's Quick Tips

- If a tooth is knocked out, it may be saved. Place the tooth in a moist, sterile gauze sponge and send it with the athlete to the dentist.

- Have the athlete stop the bleeding by placing direct pressure on the tooth socket with a sterile sponge.

Leg Cramps

Leg muscles can go into spasm and cramp, causing severe pain. Leg cramps are the result of muscle fatigue or dehydration and signal early heat exhaustion. They usually occur late in a game or practice. In my experience, the athlete has always been able to distinguish a cramp from a more serious injury, but you should make sure there is no serious injury causing the spasm before you move the leg and stretch the muscle.

Dr. Steele's Quick Tips

- Confirm that the leg cramp is not a spasm caused by a more serious injury such as a fracture.

- Feel for a muscle spasm or tight muscle.

- Treat leg cramps by stretching the affected muscle and holding the stretch for 30 seconds.
  - If the cramp is in the calf, pull the toes toward the shin while the athlete keeps the knee straight.
  - If the cramp is in the hamstring (back of thigh), straighten the knee.

- Massage the muscle until the cramp subsides.

- Don't move an athlete with a leg cramp to the sideline until the spasms subside.
- Make sure the athlete drinks fluids and shows no signs of heat exhaustion before you allow a return to play.

Wind Knocked Out

A forcible blow to the belly will literally knock the wind out of the lungs. Without air in the lungs, the athlete will gasp for air and be unable to talk. Pressure on the belly (which needs to expand) will make it harder for the athlete to reinflate his lungs. The athlete should be able to talk within 30 seconds and be experiencing no air hunger or shortness of breath within one to two minutes. If symptoms persist, evaluate for a more serious injury.

Dr. Steele's Quick Tips

- Reassure the athlete that breathing will resume normally.

- When the wind is knocked out of the athlete,
  - loosen the belt or anything restricting the belly, and
  - consider a more serious injury if the athlete is not fully recovered within one to two minutes.

PART 1

Critical Injuries

Thorough and swift evaluation may save a life or prevent serious injury to a downed athlete on the field. Assume all downed athletes have a potentially critical injury until you prove otherwise.

First determine whether the athlete is conscious. If unconscious, immediately check the *ABC*s. Is the **a**irway obstructed? Is the athlete **b**reathing? Is there **c**irculation (a pulse)? If any answer is no, call 911. You or someone trained in CPR must start CPR immediately to save the athlete.

If the athlete is conscious, assess mental status. If it is altered, the athlete may have a serious head injury or be in shock. This is a 911 emergency, and time is crucial.

Neck injuries are commonly associated with head injuries, so protect the neck while you wait for help. If the athlete is in shock, call 911 and begin treatment for shock. Never move a critically injured athlete unless he is on his back and begins vomiting. In this situation, protect the neck and roll the athlete onto his side so that he won't aspirate or choke on his vomit.

If the athlete is alert, not in shock, and mental status is normal, you can ask specific questions that pertain to the injury and complete the evaluation using the appropriate checklist. If your findings indicate a possible serious injury, immediately stop further evaluation and follow the Emergency Care Guidelines.

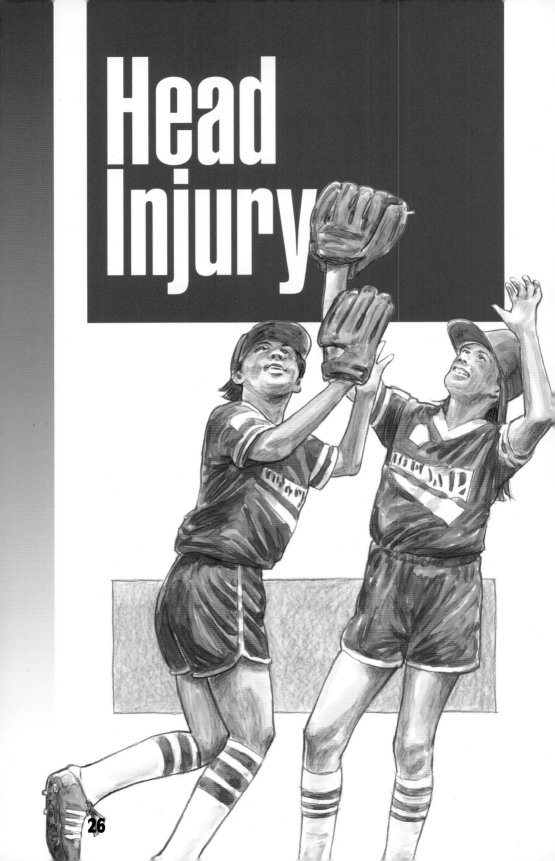

Head Injury

Time is of the essence. Head injuries are one of the most common causes of death in athletes. Any athlete who loses consciousness or shows signs of altered consciousness requires emergency care. You *must* complete a careful examination of the athlete af-

Possible Injuries

Concussion

Fractured skull

Associated neck or back injury

Bleeding into the brain

ter any suspected head injury, even when an athlete's mental state seems normal. And, because neck injuries are often associated with head injuries, it is important to stabilize and evaluate both the head and the neck. You cannot allow an athlete to return to play after a suspected head injury; only a medical professional can make this decision.

Dr. Steele's Quick Tips

- Do not remove the athlete's headgear until you are certain there is no neck injury.

- Memory loss, confusion, and belligerence are warning signs of a head injury. Ask the athlete these questions of recent memory in your evaluation:
  - "What happened?"
  - "Where are you?"
  - "What's the score?"

- Signs and symptoms of a head injury may not appear immediately; remember to recheck and closely monitor an athlete with a suspected head injury every 5 to 10 minutes.

- Take an important piece of gear away from the athlete so she cannot return to play while you're not watching.

HEAD INJURY

1 Athlete Down

▶▶▶ Don't let athlete move.
Don't move athlete.
Don't remove headgear.
Calm athlete.

2 Check for These Signs & Symptoms

▷▷▷ Unconsciousness
Obstructed airway
Abnormal breathing
No pulse or abnormal pulse
Belligerence or agitation
Confusion or nonresponsiveness
Memory loss
Shock
Severe headache
Discharge from nose or ears
Weak or numb extremities
Blurred vision
Unequal pupils
Facial paralysis
Seizures
Painful or limited neck motion
Nausea or vomiting

Any Found ▶

None Found ▶

Athlete Needs Emergency Care

▷ Call 911.
▷ Begin CPR if needed.
▷ Protect and stabilize head and neck.
▷ Treat for shock.
▷ Don't move athlete.
▷ Don't give food or water.

Assist Athlete to Sideline

▷ Reassure and calm athlete.
▷ Ask athlete if she wants to be helped to sideline.
▷ Wait until athlete can sit up and is ready to move.
▷ Help athlete slowly stand.
▷ Support athlete and walk slowly to sideline.
▷ Observe athlete's balance and general attitude.
▷ Ask athlete how she feels and what happened.

Begin Sideline Evaluation and Care ▶

HEAD INJURY

HEAD INJURY

3 | Athlete on Sideline

▷▷▷ Stop athlete from returning to game.
Assume possible neck injury.
Don't give food or water.

4 | Recheck for These Signs & Symptoms

▷ Abnormal breathing
▷ Abnormal pulse
▷ Belligerence or agitation
▷ Confusion or nonresponsiveness
▷ Memory loss
▷ Shock
▷ Severe headache
▷ Discharge from nose or ears
▷ Weak or numb extremities
▷ Blurred vision
▷ Unequal pupils
▷ Facial paralysis
▷ Seizures
▷ Painful or limited neck motion
▷ Nausea or vomiting

Any Found ▷

None Found ▷

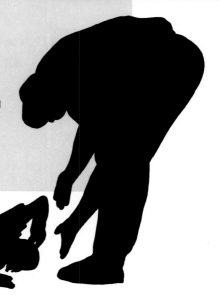

○ Athlete Needs Emergency Care

▷ Call 911.

▷ Protect and stabilize head and neck.

▷ Treat for shock.

▷ Don't give food or water.

○ Athlete Should See a Doctor Today

▷ If necessary, assist athlete home after game.

▷ Report injury to parents or guardian.

▷ Stress potential seriousness of head injuries.

▷ Encourage them to take athlete to a doctor today.

▷ Inform them athlete cannot return to play without written medical consent.

5 Athlete <u>Cannot</u> Return to Play

▷ Do not give in to pressure from parents, coaches, or players. Returning to play, even with minor symptoms, can lead to *second impact syndrome*, the sudden, unexpected death of someone who sustains a seemingly minor head injury followed by a second minor head injury. Because a number of second impact syndrome deaths have been reported, an athlete's return to play is not an option until authorized by a medical professional.

Neck Injury

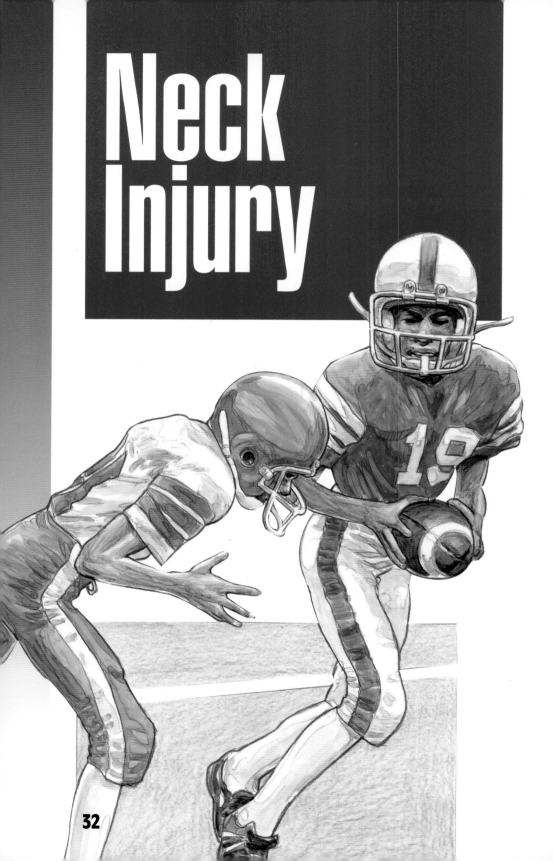

Use extreme caution when evaluating a suspected neck injury. The spinal cord passes through the vertebrae of the neck, and because damage to the spinal cord often results in paralysis, neck injuries are among the most serious injuries an athlete can sustain. Your primary responsibility is to protect the spinal cord from injury. Do not remove the athlete's headgear and do not move the neck while you evaluate the athlete. If the athlete complains of severe neck pain, reports numbness or tingling in his arms or legs, or seems unable to move, you should suspect a serious neck injury. Keep the head and neck absolutely immobile and call for emergency help.

Possible Injuries

Fractured or dislocated vertebra

Spinal cord injury

Ruptured disc

Torn ligament or muscle

Associated head injury

Dr. Steele's Quick Tips

- To prevent further injury to the spinal cord, do not remove the athlete's headgear if you suspect a neck injury.

- To protect and stabilize an athlete's head and neck during your evaluation, kneel on the ground near his head, place your hands on each side of his head and neck, and hold his head gently but securely between your hands.

- When evaluating for a neck injury, give this four-extremity test. Ask the athlete to
  - grip with his right hand, then lift his right arm,
  - grip with his left hand, then lift his left arm,
  - wiggle his right foot, then lift his right leg, and
  - wiggle his left foot, then lift his left leg.

NECK INJURY

1 Athlete Down

▷ Don't let athlete move.
▷ Don't move athlete.
▷ Don't remove headgear.
▷ Calm athlete.

2 Check for These Signs & Symptoms

▷ Unconsciousness
▷ Obstructed airway
▷ Abnormal breathing
▷ No pulse or abnormal pulse
▷ Shock
▷ Severe neck pain
▷ Fails four-extremity test
▷ Weak, tingling, or numb extremities
▷ Localized neck tenderness
▷ Painful or limited neck motion

Any Found ▷

None Found ▷

Athlete Needs Emergency Care

▷ Call 911.
▷ Begin CPR if needed.
▷ Protect and stabilize head and neck.
▷ Treat for shock.
▷ Don't move athlete.
▷ Don't give food or water.

Assist Athlete to Sideline

▷ Reassure and calm athlete.
▷ Ask athlete if he wants to be helped to sideline.
▷ Wait until athlete can sit up and is ready to move.
▷ Help athlete slowly stand.
▷ Support athlete and walk slowly to sideline.
▷ Observe athlete's balance and general attitude.
▷ Ask athlete how he feels and what happened.

Begin Sideline Evaluation and Care

NECK INJURY

NECK INJURY

3 Athlete on Sideline

▷▷▷ Stop athlete from returning to game.
Assume possible head injury.
Don't give food or water.

4 Recheck for These Signs & Symptoms

▷ Abnormal breathing
▷ Abnormal pulse
▷ Shock
▷ Severe neck pain
▷ Fails four-extremity test
▷ Weak, tingling, or numb extremities
▷ Localized neck tenderness
▷ Painful or limited neck motion

Any Found ▷

None Found ▷

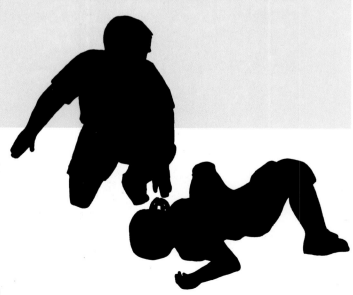

Athlete Needs Emergency Care

▷ Call 911.

▷ Protect and stabilize head and neck.

▷ Treat for shock.

▷ Don't give food or water.

Athlete Should See a Doctor Today

▷ If necessary, assist athlete home after game.

▷ Report injury to parents or guardian.

▷ Stress potential seriousness of neck injuries.

▷ Encourage them to take athlete to a doctor today.

▷ Inform them athlete cannot return to play without written medical consent.

5 Athlete <u>Cannot</u> Return to Play

▷ Do not give in to pressure from parents, coaches, or players. Because even minor neck injuries can damage the spinal cord, returning the athlete to the game is not an option until authorized by a medical professional.

NECK INJURY

Back Injury

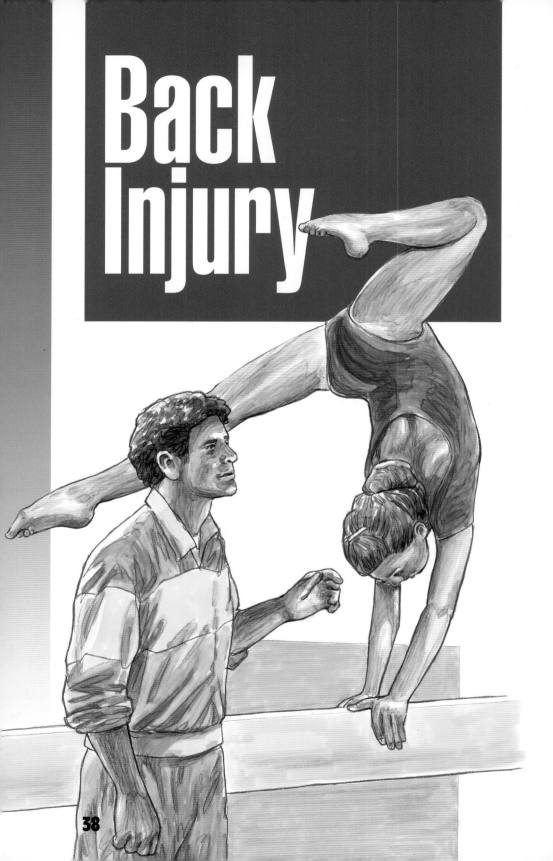

Never carry an athlete with a suspected back injury off the field. Like neck injuries, back injuries should be handled with extreme caution. If handled incorrectly, a fractured or dislocated vertebra could result in nerve or spinal cord damage. Therefore, a thorough but cautious evaluation of the back should be done on-field before assisting the athlete to the sideline. An athlete's return to play after a back injury should only be authorized by a medical professional.

Possible Injuries

Fractured vertebra

Spinal cord injury

Ruptured disc

Torn ligament or muscle

Associated head or neck injury

Dr. Steele's Quick Tips

- Consider any athlete who reports feeling a tingling sensation in her legs, even if it was momentary, to have a potentially serious back injury.

- If you suspect a back injury has occurred, give this two-extremity test. Ask the athlete to
  - wiggle her right foot, then lift her right leg and
  - wiggle her left foot, then lift her left leg.

- If there are no other signs or symptoms, check for localized tenderness along the spine. Start between the shoulder blades, pressing gently against each vertebra, and progress down to the lower back. Tenderness at any vertebra indicates a possible fracture. Keep the athlete still and call for professional help.

BACK INJURY

1   Athlete Down

▶ Don't let athlete move.
▶ Don't move athlete.
▶ Calm athlete.

2   Check for These Signs & Symptoms

▶ Unconsciousness
▶ Obstructed airway
▶ Abnormal breathing
▶ No pulse or abnormal pulse
▶ Shock
▶ Severe back pain
▶ Fails two-extremity test
▶ Weak, tingling, or numb legs or feet
▶ Localized back tenderness
▶ Painful or limited back motion

Any Found ▶

None Found ▶

Athlete Needs Emergency Care

▷ Call 911.
▷ Begin CPR if needed.
▷ Protect and stabilize neck and spine.
▷ Treat for shock.
▷ Don't move athlete.
▷ Don't give food or water.

Assist Athlete to Sideline

▷ Reassure and calm athlete.
▷ Ask athlete if she wants to be helped to sideline.
▷ Wait until athlete can sit up and is ready to move.
▷ Help athlete slowly stand.
▷ Support athlete and walk slowly to sideline.
▷ Observe athlete's balance and general attitude.
▷ Ask athlete how she feels and what happened.

Begin Sideline Evaluation and Care

BACK INJURY

3 Athlete on Sideline

▷▷▷ Stop athlete from returning to game.
Assume possible spinal injury.
Don't give food or water.

4 Recheck for These Signs & Symptoms

▷▷▷▷▷▷▷▷ Abnormal breathing
Abnormal pulse
Shock
Severe back pain
Fails two-extremity test
Weak, tingling, or numb legs or feet
Localized back tenderness
Painful or limited back motion

Any Found ▷

None Found ▷

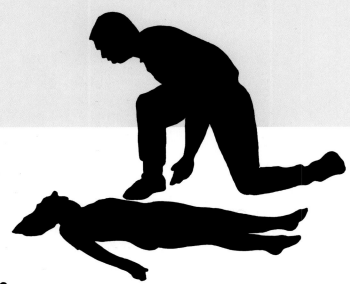

Athlete Needs Emergency Care

▶ Call 911.

▶ Protect and stabilize neck and spine.

▶ Treat for shock.

▶ Don't give food or water.

Athlete Should See a Doctor Today

▶ If necessary, assist athlete home after game.

▶ Report injury to parents or guardian.

▶ Stress potential seriousness of back injuries.

▶ Encourage them to take athlete to a doctor today.

▶ Inform them athlete cannot return to play without written medical consent.

5 Athlete <u>Cannot</u> Return to Play

▶ Returning the athlete to play can only be authorized by a medical professional because the risk of spinal cord injury is too great. Never give in to pressure from parents, coaches, or players.

BACK INJURY

Heat Stroke

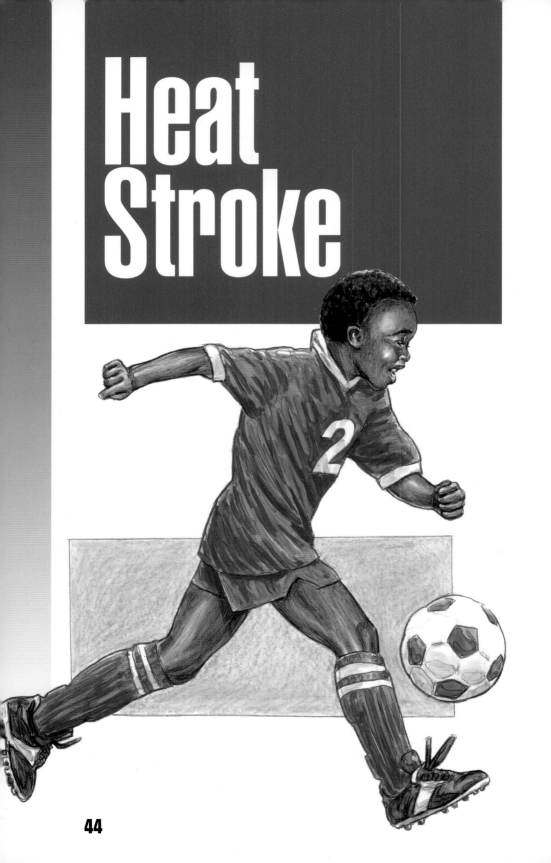

Heat stroke may cause death if not recognized and treated immediately. Heat stroke occurs when an athlete's internal temperature control system fails, causing his body temperature to rise to dangerous levels. Heat exhaustion is a precursor to heat stroke. An athlete who develops cramps, weakness, fatigue, and nausea is exhibiting signs of heat exhaustion. Fortunately, heat stroke and heat exhaustion are preventable. Heat emergencies usually occur under conditions of extreme heat and humidity, so overweight, unconditioned, or overdressed athletes are at high risk, especially during preseason training. Be sure to allow your athletes frequent water breaks.

Dr. Steele's Quick Tips

- Because the sensation of being thirsty lags behind the body's actual physical need for water, you must encourage your athletes to drink even when they are not thirsty.

- Do not allow your athletes to take salt tablets. Instead, provide them with electrolyte sports drinks.

- An athlete who develops cramps, weakness, fatigue, and nausea is exhibiting signs of heat exhaustion (a precursor to heat stroke) and should be made to rest in the shade and drink fluids to cool off.

- Remember, the athlete may have been sweating, so his skin may at first seem wet or clammy rather than dry.

- When treating a heat stroke victim for shock, keep the athlete cool rather than warm.

HEAT STROKE

1 Athlete Down

▷▷▷ Don't let athlete move.
Don't move unconscious athlete.
Move conscious athlete to shade.
Calm athlete.

2 Check for These Signs & Symptoms

▷ Unconsciousness
▷ Obstructed airway
▷ Abnormal breathing
▷ No pulse or abnormal pulse
▷ Red, hot, and dry skin
▷ Very small pupils
▷ Very high body temperature
▷ No sweating
▷ Belligerence or agitation
▷ Confusion or nonresponsiveness
▷ Memory loss
▷ Shock

Any Found ▷

None Found ▷

Athlete Needs Emergency Care

▷ Call 911.
▷ Begin CPR if needed.
▷ Treat for shock.
▷ Remove athlete's excess clothing.
▷ Douse athlete with cold water.
▷ Fan athlete with towels.

Assist Athlete to Sideline

▷ Reassure and calm athlete.
▷ Ask athlete if he wants to be helped to sideline.
▷ Wait until athlete can sit up and is ready to move.
▷ Help athlete slowly stand.
▷ Support athlete and walk slowly to sideline.
▷ Observe athlete's skin tone and general attitude.
▷ Ask athlete if he feels hot and what happened.

Begin Sideline Evaluation and Care

HEAT STROKE

3 Athlete on Sideline

▷▷▷ Stop athlete from returning to game.
Keep athlete still.
Keep athlete in shade.

4 Recheck for These Signs & Symptoms

▷ Abnormal breathing
▷ Abnormal pulse
▷ Red, hot, and dry skin
▷ Very small pupils
▷ Very high body temperature
▷ No sweating
▷ Belligerence or agitation
▷ Confusion or nonresponsiveness
▷ Memory loss
▷ Shock

Any Found ▷

None Found ▷

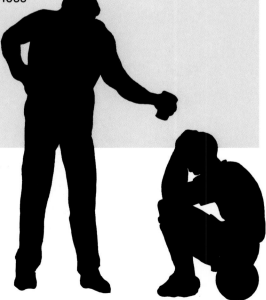

Athlete Needs Emergency Care

Call 911.

Treat for shock.

Remove athlete's excess clothing.

Douse athlete with cold water.

Fan athlete with towels.

Athlete Should See a Doctor Today

Have athlete rest in the shade and drink fluids.

If necessary, assist athlete home after game.

Report heat emergency to parents or guardian.

Stress potential seriousness of heat stroke.

Encourage them to take athlete to a doctor today.

Inform them athlete cannot return to play without written medical consent.

5 Athlete <u>Cannot</u> Return to Play

As with all other life-threatening injuries, only a medical professional should authorize an athlete's return to play after heat stroke. Even if no symptoms of heat stroke or other injury are found, an athlete should not return to play after collapsing on the field. He may be suffering from heat exhaustion and dehydration, and it may take a day or two for him to recover.

PART 2

Internal Organ Injuries

After you have established that the athlete is conscious, alert, breathing, and has not sustained any injury to the head, neck, or spine, you may proceed to evaluate the injured abdomen or chest. Blunt trauma to the trunk of the body can cause injuries to the chest or abdomen that may not be apparent. These injuries are often associated with breathing problems or serious internal bleeding, and they can be fatal.

Shock may be the first sign of injury. Signs of shock include rapid pulse, profuse sweating, cool and clammy skin, dizziness, paleness, and nausea or vomiting.

The serious signs and symptoms associated with injuries to internal organs may be delayed 10 to 20 minutes or longer. Therefore, do not assume that everything is fine even when the athlete seems to recover quickly. As with all critical injuries, reexamination and a high degree of suspicion are essential.

Use the following checklists to evaluate for internal injuries. If your findings indicate a possible serious injury, immediately stop further evaluation and follow the Emergency Care Guidelines.

Chest Injury

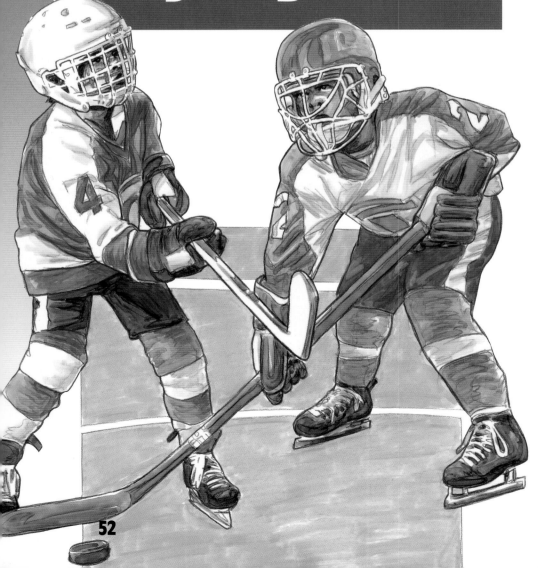

M ost chest injuries are caused by a blunt blow to the area, and there are few or no signs of external trauma. This blow may fracture ribs, which in turn could puncture a lung, causing it to collapse or fill with blood. Both are poten-

tially fatal situations. Labored or abnormal breathing and severe pain in the ribs, breastbone, or top of the shoulder are indications of a serious chest injury; loosen the athlete's clothing to ease breathing and wait for emergency help.

Another less serious injury that might be confused with a chest injury can occur when a blow to the stomach literally knocks the air out of an athlete, making it difficult for him to talk for about 15 seconds until he can catch his breath. If the athlete cannot talk and breathe normally within one to two minutes, evaluate for a more serious chest injury.

Dr. Steele's Quick Tips

- You can assume a serious chest injury has occurred if
  - the athlete is having breathing difficulty or pain with breathing, or
  - the athlete feels extreme pain over the ribs, breastbone, or top of the shoulder.
- When an athlete gets his wind knocked out, loosen the belt or other clothing restricting the belly to allow the lungs to reinflate.

CHEST INJURY

1 Athlete Down

▸▸▸ Don't let athlete move.
Don't move athlete.
Calm athlete.

2 Check for These Signs & Symptoms

▸▸▸ Labored breathing
Fast or shallow breathing
Shortness of breath
Severe pain at ribs, breastbone, or top of shoulder
Pain increases with breathing
Shock

Any Found ▸

None Found ▸

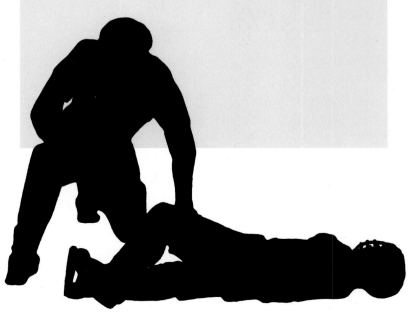

Athlete Needs Emergency Care

Call 911.

Loosen clothing to ease breathing.

Treat for shock.

Don't move athlete.

Don't give food or water.

Assist Athlete to Sideline

Reassure and calm athlete.

Allow athlete to catch his breath.

Ask athlete if he wants to be helped to sideline.

Wait until athlete can sit up and is ready to move.

Help athlete slowly stand.

Support athlete and walk slowly to sideline.

Observe athlete's breathing and general attitude.

Ask athlete how he feels.

Begin Sideline Evaluation and Care

CHEST INJURY

CHEST INJURY

3 Athlete on Sideline

▷ Stop athlete from returning to game.
▷ Remove athletic gear.

4 Recheck for These Signs & Symptoms

▷ Labored breathing
▷ Fast or shallow breathing
▷ Shortness of breath
▷ Severe pain at ribs, breastbone, or top of shoulder
▷ Pain increases with breathing
▷ Shock

Any Found ▷

None Found ▷

5 Check for These Signs & Symptoms

▷ Localized tenderness on ribs or breastbone
▷ Painful ribs with motion

Any Found ▷

None Found ▷

Athlete Needs Emergency Care

▷ Call 911.

▷ Loosen clothing to ease breathing.

▷ Treat for shock.

▷ Don't give food or water.

Athlete Should See a Doctor Today

▷ If necessary, assist athlete home after game.

▷ Report injury to parents or guardian.

▷ Stress potential seriousness of chest injuries.

▷ Encourage them to take athlete to a doctor today.

▷ Inform them athlete cannot return to play without written medical consent.

Athlete Can Return to Play

▷ If reevaluation is normal after athlete sits for 5 to 10 minutes

▷ If athlete only had his wind knocked out

▷ If athlete is not in pain

▷ If athlete can breathe normally

▷ If athlete wants to return to play

CHEST INJURY

57

Abdominal Injury

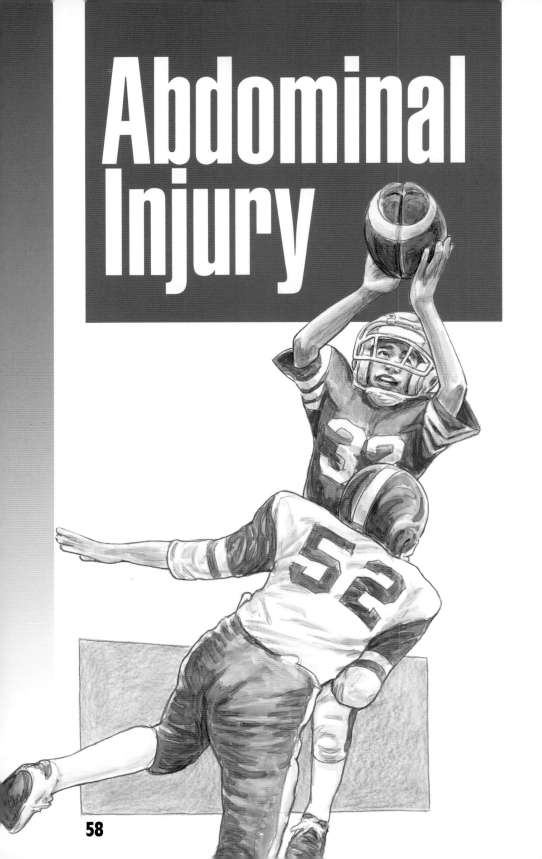

Never assume that an abdominal injury is minor. A blow to the abdominal area can tear an organ, causing internal bleeding. Like chest injuries, there will be no external signs of injury. If internal bleeding is rapid, the ath-

Possible Injuries

Ruptured internal organ

Bruised abdominal muscle

Testicle injury

lete will quickly report pain in the abdomen and across the top of the shoulder and show signs of blood loss and shock. However, if the bleeding is very slow, these signs may not occur for several minutes to several hours after the injury. It is critical that you reevaluate the athlete often after he is on the sideline and educate his parents or guardian about what signs or symptoms they should look for in the hours after the injury.

A testicle injury is one type of blunt trauma injury that, while painful, is usually not serious. However, a blow may occasionally cause a testicle to rupture, so treat severe, persisting pain as a symptom of a more serious injury.

Dr. Steele's Quick Tips

■ Athletes with abdominal injuries, even serious ones, usually do not show signs of injury immediately. Continue to monitor a sidelined athlete with a suspected abdominal injury and recheck his condition every 5 to 10 minutes.

■ If you suspect an athlete might have an abdominal injury, monitor the athlete for signs of shock by checking for

■ a pulse that remains greater than 120 beats per minute,
■ profuse sweating,
■ cool, clammy skin,
■ dizziness,
■ paleness, and
■ nausea or vomiting.

59

ABDOMINAL INJURY

1 Athlete Down

▶▶ Don't let athlete move.
▶ Don't move athlete.
▶ Calm athlete.

2 Check for These Signs & Symptoms

▶▶ Severe abdominal pain or tenderness
▶ Severe pain at top of shoulder
▶ Pain increases with breathing
▶ Shock

Any Found ▶

None Found ▶

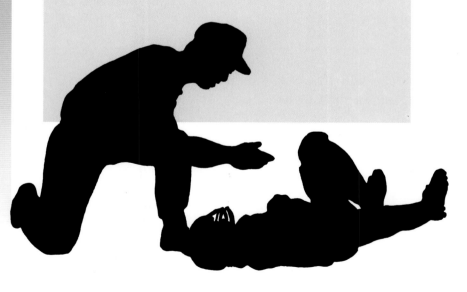

Athlete Needs Emergency Care

Call 911.

Loosen clothing to ease pressure on abdomen.

Treat for shock.

Don't move athlete.

Don't give food or water.

Assist Athlete to Sideline

Reassure and calm athlete.

Ask athlete if he wants to be helped to sideline.

Wait until athlete can sit up and is ready to move.

Help athlete slowly stand.

Support athlete and walk slowly to sideline.

Observe athlete's general attitude.

Ask athlete how he feels.

Begin Sideline Evaluation and Care ▶

ABDOMINAL INJURY

ABDOMINAL INJURY

3 Athlete on Sideline

▷▷ Stop athlete from returning to game.
Remove athletic gear.

4 Recheck for These Signs & Symptoms

▷▷▷▷ Severe abdominal pain or tenderness

Any Found ▷

Severe pain at top of shoulder
Pain increases with breathing

None Found ▷

Shock

Athlete Needs Emergency Care

▷ Call 911.

▷ Loosen clothing to ease pressure on abdomen.

▷ Treat for shock.

▷ Don't give food or water.

Athlete Should See a Doctor Today

▷ If necessary, assist athlete home after game.

▷ Report injury to parents or guardian.

▷ Stress potential seriousness of abdominal injuries.

▷ Describe serious and potentially delayed signs and symptoms to look for, including blood in urine.

▷ Encourage them to take athlete to a doctor today.

▷ Inform them athlete cannot return to play without written medical consent.

5 Athlete <u>Cannot</u> Return to Play

▷ Because the effects of an abdominal injury may occur several minutes or hours after the injury itself, returning a seemingly healthy athlete immediately to play could cause more damage. Even if the injury seems minor, only a medical professional can make the decision to return the athlete to play.

PART 3

Facial Injuries

After you have established that the athlete is conscious, alert, breathing, and has not sustained any injury to the head, neck, spine, or internal organs, you may proceed to evaluate the facial injury. A hard blow to the face may cause an injury to the eye, nose, jaw, or facial bones. When associated with breathing problems, any facial, head, neck, or jaw injury can be a threat to life. Even a severe nosebleed can put an athlete with a blood-clotting disorder at risk. Fortunately, most facial injuries are not serious, but improper handling of eye, nose, or jaw injuries can result in permanent damage. Use the following checklists for each specific injury. If your findings indicate a possible serious injury, immediately stop further evaluation and follow the Emergency Care Guidelines.

Eye Injury

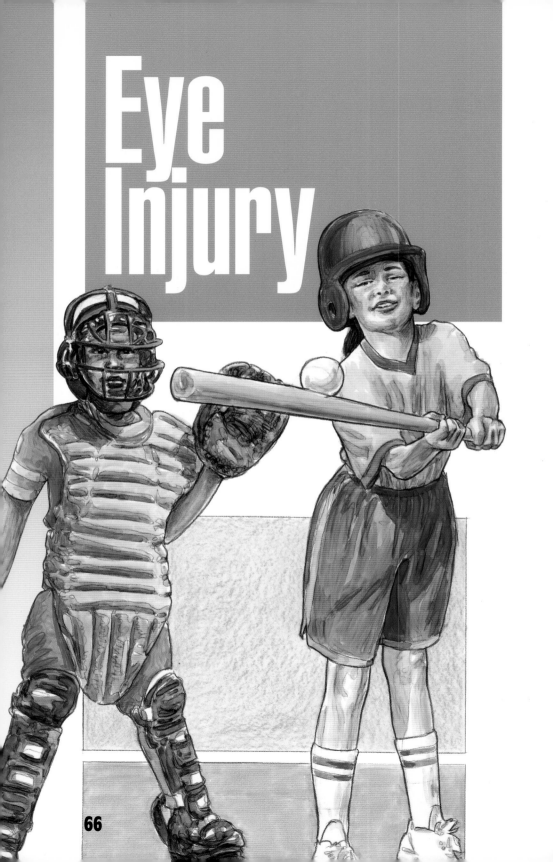

Always evaluate any athlete with an eye injury for an associated head or neck injury. Eye injuries include cuts on and around the eye and blunt injuries to both the eye and the surrounding bone. Loss of vision, severe pain or tenderness, and cuts around the eye require immediate medical attention. Remember also that memory loss, confusion, belligerence, paralyzed or weak extremities, and painful neck motion are all indications of a serious head or neck injury. If there is no sign of a head or neck injury, you may decide to transport the athlete to a medical facility yourself; however, if you're unsure of the seriousness of the injury, call for emergency help.

Possible Injuries

Detached retina

Lacerated eye

Bleeding inside eye

Fracture of bone around eye

Foreign body in eye

Scratched eye surface

Associated head or neck injury

Dr. Steele's Quick Tips

- While you are evaluating the eye, don't
  - remove the athlete's contact lenses,
  - wash the eye, or
  - allow the athlete to rub or press her eye.

- Because the eyes travel as a unit, to protect and prevent movement of the injured eye you must
  - have the athlete close her eyes,
  - place a gauze sponge over the injured eye, and
  - tape both eyes shut.

1 Athlete Down

▷▷▷ Don't move athlete.
Don't let athlete rub eye.
Calm athlete.

2 Check for These Signs & Symptoms

▷▷▷▷▷▷ Loss of or blurred vision
Bleeding in or around eye
Severe pain
Extreme tenderness around eye
Numbness below eye
Foreign object in eye
Unequal pupils

Any Found ▷

None Found ▷

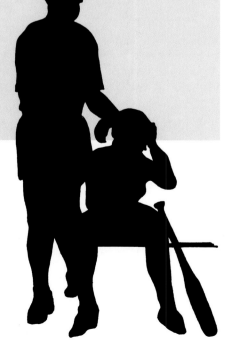

Athlete Needs Emergency Care

Call 911 or transport athlete to medical facility.

Don't remove contact lenses.

Protect and immobilize eye.

Don't give food or water.

Assist Athlete to Sideline

Reassure and calm athlete.

Ask athlete if she wants to be helped to sideline.

Wait until athlete can sit up and is ready to move.

Help athlete slowly stand.

Support athlete and walk slowly to sideline.

Observe athlete's general attitude.

Ask athlete how she feels.

Begin Sideline Evaluation and Care

EYE INJURY

EYE INJURY

3 Athlete on Sideline

▷▷▷ Stop athlete from returning to game.
Don't let athlete rub eye.
Move athlete to a well-lit area.

4 Recheck for These Signs & Symptoms

▷▷▷▷▷▷▷ Loss of or blurred vision
Bleeding in or around eye
Severe pain   **Any Found** ▷
Extreme tenderness around eye
Numbness below eye   **None Found** ▷
Foreign object in eye
Unequal pupils

Athlete Needs Emergency Care

Call 911 or transport athlete to medical facility.

Don't remove contact lenses.

Protect and immobilize eye.

Don't give food or water.

Athlete Should See a Doctor Today

If necessary, assist athlete home after game.

Report injury to parents or guardian.

Stress potential seriousness of eye injuries.

Encourage them to take athlete to a doctor today.

Inform them athlete cannot return to play without written medical consent.

5 Athlete <u>Cannot</u> Return to Play

Eye injuries can be more serious than they appear. Do not give in to pressure from parents, coaches, or players. An athlete's return to play is not an option until authorized by a medical professional.

EYE INJURY

Nose Injury

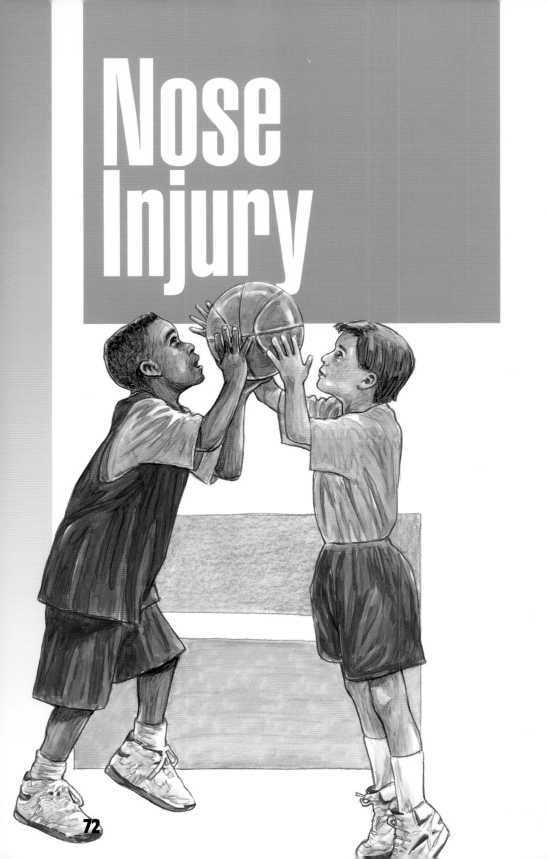

The most common nose injuries are fractured or bloody noses. Unless nose injuries are associated with a head or neck injury, which is rare, it is usually possible for you to transport the athlete to a medical facility yourself. However,

Fractured nose

Bloody nose

Associated head or neck injury

don't hesitate to call for emergency help in these circumstances: Clear fluid instead of blood is coming out of the nose, there are signs of a head or neck injury, you can't stop the bleeding (a possibility for athletes with blood-clotting disorders or a history of severe nosebleeds), or you aren't sure of the seriousness of the injury.

Dr. Steele's Quick Tips

- When treating a bloody nose,
  - avoid tilting the athlete's head back, which will cause blood to run down the athlete's throat; and
  - avoid packing gauze into the athlete's nose, because it could become lodged in the throat.

  Instead, tilt the athlete's head forward and apply pressure and ice to the nose.

- Make sure an athlete suffering from significant swelling, deformity, or pain sees a medical professional promptly.

NOSE INJURY

1 Athlete Down

Don't move athlete.
Don't let athlete tilt head back.
Calm athlete.

2 Check for These Signs & Symptoms

Clear fluid coming out of nose
Rapid, unstoppable bleeding

Any Found ▷

None Found ▷

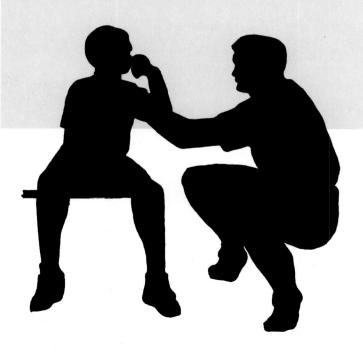

Athlete Needs Emergency Care

▷ Call 911 or transport athlete to medical facility.

▷ Tilt head forward and apply gauze sponge and ice to nose.

▷ Don't give food or water.

Assist Athlete to Sideline

▷ Reassure and calm athlete.

▷ Ask athlete if he wants to be helped to sideline.

▷ Wait until athlete can sit up and is ready to move.

▷ Help athlete slowly stand.

▷ Support athlete and walk slowly to sideline.

▷ Observe athlete's general attitude.

▷ Ask athlete how he feels.

Begin Sideline Evaluation and Care ▶

NOSE INJURY

NOSE INJURY

3 Athlete on Sideline

Stop athlete from returning to game.
Don't let athlete tilt head back.

4 Recheck for These Signs & Symptoms

Clear fluid coming out of nose
Rapid, unstoppable bleeding

Any Found

None Found

5 Check for These Signs & Symptoms

Deformed nose
Swelling
Severe pain
Grating bones
Localized tenderness

Any Found

None Found

Athlete Needs Emergency Care

▷ Call 911 or transport athlete to medical facility.

▷ Tilt head forward and apply gauze sponge and ice to nose.

▷ Don't give food or water.

Athlete Should See a Doctor Today

▷ If necessary, assist athlete home after game.

▷ Report injury to parents or guardian.

▷ Stress potential seriousness of nose injuries.

▷ Encourage them to take athlete to a doctor today.

▷ Inform them athlete cannot return to play without written medical consent.

Athlete Can Return to Play

▷ If reevaluation is normal after athlete sits for 5 to 10 minutes

▷ If bleeding stops promptly

▷ If athlete is not in pain

▷ If athlete wants to return to play

NOSE INJURY

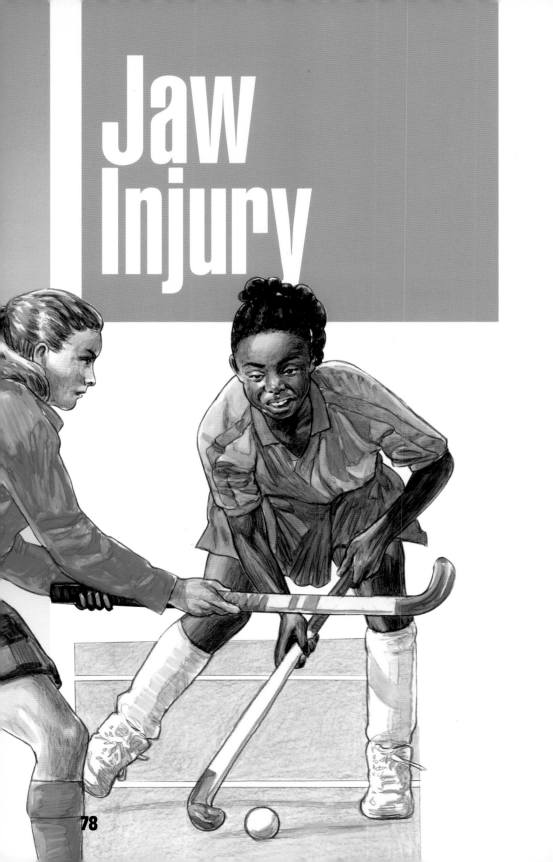

Jaw
Injury

A hard blow to the mouth may fracture an athlete's jaw, dislodge or break teeth, and cause an associated head or neck injury. If the athlete is having difficulty breathing or speaking, then blood, teeth, or vomit may be obstructing the airway and you need to clear it immediately. Call for help if the athlete is showing signs and symptoms of a head or neck injury, is experiencing severe pain or breathing problems, or is unable to open or close her mouth. You can transport the athlete to a medical facility or dentist yourself if a careful evaluation reveals that the injury resulted only in broken or missing teeth.

Possible Injuries

Fractured jaw

Broken or missing teeth

Associated head or neck injury

Dr. Steele's Quick Tips

- Follow these steps to clear the athlete's airway:
  - If the athlete is on her back and vomiting, roll her onto her side while protecting the neck.
  - If the athlete is conscious and you have ruled out a neck injury, lean her forward to let blood, teeth, and vomit drain out of the mouth rather than into the back of the throat.
- Remove any broken or loose teeth and save them in a moist, sterile sponge. Using the athlete's own saliva to moisten the sponge is excellent.

JAW INJURY

1 Athlete Down

▼▼▼ Don't let athlete move.
Don't move athlete.
Calm athlete.

2 Check for These Signs & Symptoms

▼▼▼▼▼ Noisy or difficult breathing
Difficulty talking
Severe pain
Inability to open or close mouth
Deformed jaw

Any Found ▷

None Found ▷

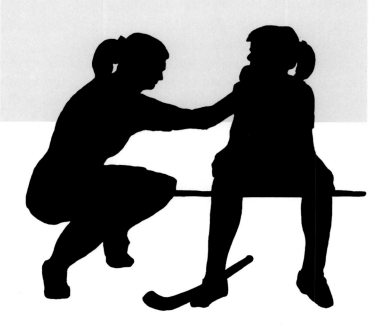

Athlete Needs Emergency Care

▷▷▷ Call 911 or transport athlete to medical facility.

▷▷▷ Roll athlete onto side or lean athlete forward to keep airway clear.

▷▷▷ Apply ice to jaw.

▷▷▷ Don't give food or water.

 ## Assist Athlete to Sideline

▷ Reassure and calm athlete.

▷ Ask athlete if she wants to be helped to sideline.

▷ Wait until athlete can sit up and is ready to move.

▷ Help athlete slowly stand.

▷ Support athlete and walk slowly to sideline.

▷ Observe athlete's general attitude.

▷ Ask athlete how she feels.

Begin Sideline Evaluation and Care ▶

JAW INJURY

3 Athlete on Sideline

▶ Stop athlete from returning to game.
▶ Don't let athlete tilt head back.

4 Recheck for These Signs & Symptoms

▶ Noisy or difficult breathing
▶ Difficulty talking   **Any Found** ▶
▶ Severe pain
▶ Inability to open or close mouth   **None Found** ▶
▶ Deformed jaw

5 Check for These Signs & Symptoms

▶ Localized tenderness around jaw   **Any Found** ▶
▶ Difficulty opening and closing
  mouth   **None Found** ▶
▶ Swelling

Athlete Needs Emergency Care

▷ Call 911 or transport athlete to medical facility.

▷ Lean athlete forward to keep airway clear.

▷ Apply ice to jaw.

▷ Don't give food or water.

Athlete Should See a Doctor Today

▷ If necessary, assist athlete home after game.

▷ Report injury to parents or guardian.

▷ Stress potential seriousness of jaw injuries.

▷ Encourage them to take athlete to a doctor today.

▷ Inform them athlete cannot return to play without written medical consent.

Athlete Can Return to Play

▷ If reevaluation is normal after athlete sits for 5 to 10 minutes

▷ If athlete completely opens and closes mouth without pain

▷ If athlete wants to return to play

PART 4

Extremity Injuries

After establishing that the athlete is conscious, alert, breathing, and has not sustained any injury to the head, neck, spine, or internal organs, you may evaluate the injured extremity. Extremity injuries, except when there is severe bleeding, usually are not life threatening. However, if they are not handled properly, you risk permanent damage to the extremity and occasionally loss of the limb because the nerves and arteries run very close to the bones and joints and are easily damaged in these injuries. Shock usually is not associated with extremity injuries but, as with all serious injuries, you should be alert for signs of shock.

Use the following checklists for extremity injuries, and be sure to include the Eight Important Checks in your evaluation. Athletes with a serious extremity injury should not be moved or assisted from the field; instead refer to the Emergency Care Guidelines and wait for trained medical assistance. However, athletes with minor injuries usually *can* be assisted from the field. In these instances, use the PRICE Guidelines in treatment, and return the athlete to play only if she meets all the criteria outlined in the checklists. Athletes who do not return to play should see a medical professional for further evaluation.

Shoulder Injury

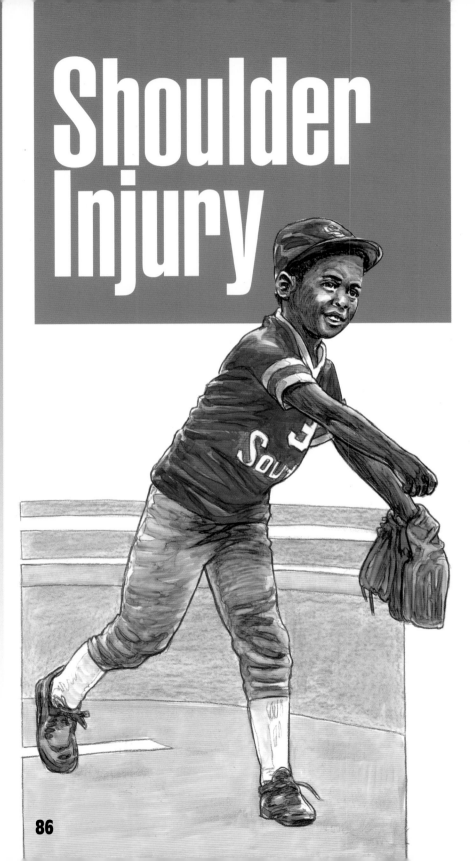

Serious shoulder injuries include fractures to the clavicle (collarbone) or upper arm (humerus), dislocations of the shoulder, and separations (collarbone from shoulder blade). Major nerves and blood vessels are very close to the bones and can be injured. Severe pain or deformity are the usual signs of serious injury. In these cases, wait for emergency help.

Many shoulder injuries are not serious. Checking range of motion is often the best way to determine the severity of the injury. Have the athlete reach over the top of his head and touch his opposite ear. If he can do this without pain, a serious shoulder injury is unlikely. If the injury does not appear to be serious, you can decide to transport the athlete to a medical facility yourself.

Dr. Steele's Quick Tips

- When treating a severe shoulder injury, call for emergency help and stabilize the shoulder where it lies. Do not attempt to straighten any deformity or move the athlete to the sideline.

- Pain across the top of the shoulder might be mistaken for a neck injury. If you think the athlete might also have suffered a neck injury, check for neck pain or tenderness and extremity numbness or paralysis to be sure.

- Check for painful or limited motion by asking the athlete to
  - reach over his head with the injured arm to touch the opposite ear or
  - move his arm outward against resistance.

SHOULDER INJURY

1 Athlete Down

▷▷▷▷ Don't let athlete move.
Don't move athlete.
Don't move or rotate shoulder.
Calm athlete.

2 Check for These Signs & Symptoms

▷▷▷▷▷▷▷▷▷ Severe pain
Deformity
Compound fracture or puncture wound
Grating bones
Numb forearm or hand
No pulse at wrist
Weak elbow or hand
Severe localized tenderness
Painful range of motion

Any Found ▷

None Found ▷

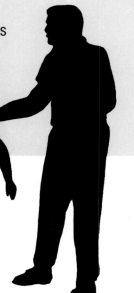

Athlete Needs Emergency Care

Call 911 or transport athlete to medical facility.
Don't try to straighten a deformity.
Cover all wounds.
Protect and stabilize shoulder.
Don't give food or water.

Assist Athlete to Sideline

Reassure and calm athlete.
Ask athlete if he wants to be helped to sideline.
Wait until athlete can sit up and is ready to move.
Stabilize athlete's arm against his body.
Help athlete slowly stand.
Support athlete and walk slowly to sideline.
Observe athlete's general attitude.
Ask athlete how he feels.

Begin Sideline Evaluation and Care

3 Athlete on Sideline

▷▷ Stop athlete from returning to game.
▷▷ Remove athletic gear, starting with uninjured arm.

4 Recheck for These Signs & Symptoms

▷▷ Severe pain
▷▷ Deformity
▷▷ Compound fracture or puncture wound
▷▷ Grating bones
▷▷ Numb forearm or hand
▷▷ No pulse at wrist
▷▷ Weak elbow or hand
▷▷ Severe localized tenderness
▷▷ Painful range of motion

Any Found ▷

None Found ▷

5 Check for These Signs & Symptoms

▷▷ Swelling
▷▷ Localized tenderness
▷▷ Limited range of motion
▷▷ Weak shoulder

Any Found ▷

None Found ▷

Athlete Needs Emergency Care

▷ Call 911 or transport athlete to medical facility.

▷ Cover all wounds.

▷ Protect and stabilize shoulder.

▷ Don't give food or water.

Athlete Should See a Doctor Today

▷ Follow PRICE Guidelines: protect, rest, ice, compress, elevate.

▷ If necessary, assist athlete home after game.

▷ Report injury to parents or guardian.

▷ Stress potential seriousness of shoulder injuries.

▷ Encourage them to take athlete to a doctor today.

▷ Inform them athlete cannot return to play without written medical consent.

Athlete Can Return to Play

▷ If reevaluation is normal after athlete sits for 5 to 10 minutes

▷ If athlete has full, pain-free range of motion

▷ If athlete has normal strength

▷ If athlete performs push-ups without pain

▷ If athlete wants to return to play

Elbow Injury

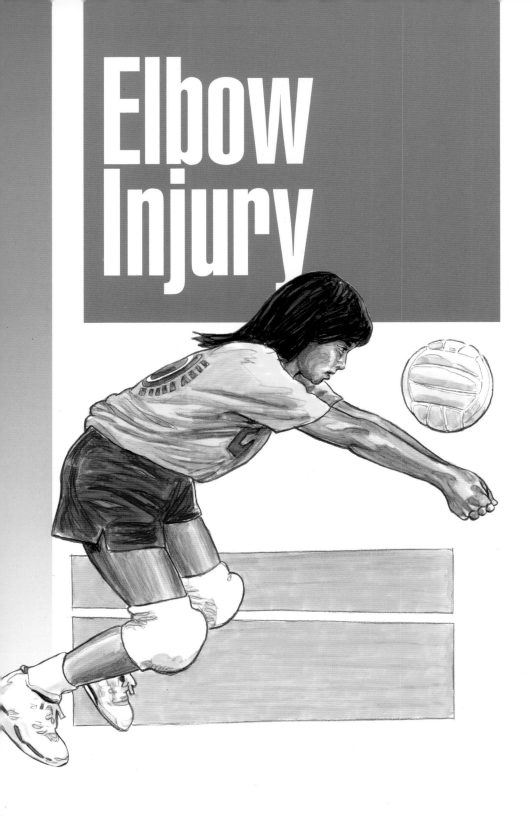

Elbow injuries can be the most serious upper extremity injury. One major artery and three major nerves run close to the bone and can be damaged by a severe elbow injury. Deformity and severe pain are warning signs that the nerves and the artery may be in danger. In this situation, do not move the elbow, but splint it in the position in which it lies and get emergency help to move the athlete and transport her to the hospital.

Possible Injuries

Fractured or dislocated elbow

Fracture above
or below the elbow

Torn ligament

Bruised elbow

Falls onto an outstretched hand may transmit enough force to the elbow to fracture it. Often an elbow injury is not overly painful, but do not be misled into thinking there is no problem. You can usually determine subtle fractures by carefully checking to make sure that the elbow can be straightened fully and that the forearm can be rotated fully. Loss of motion generally indicates a fracture. You may transport athletes with less serious injuries to a medical facility yourself.

Dr. Steele's Quick Tips

■ When treating a severe elbow injury, call for emergency help and splint the elbow where it lies. Do not attempt to straighten any deformity or move the athlete to the sideline.

■ Check for painful or limited motion by asking the athlete to
  ■ bend her injured elbow to touch her shoulder or completely straighten the injured elbow and
  ■ turn her palm up and down completely.

ELBOW INJURY

1 Athlete Down

▷▷▷ Don't let athlete move.
Don't move athlete.
Don't straighten or bend elbow.
Calm athlete.

2 Check for These Signs & Symptoms

▷▷▷ Severe pain
Deformity
Compound fracture or puncture wound
Grating bones
Numb hand
No pulse at wrist
Weak hand
Severe localized tenderness
Painful range of motion

Any Found ▷

None Found ▷

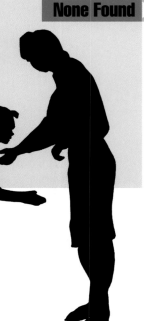

Athlete Needs Emergency Care

▷ Call 911 or transport athlete to medical facility.
▷ Don't try to straighten a deformity.
▷ Cover all wounds.
▷ Splint elbow.
▷ Don't give food or water.

 Assist Athlete to Sideline

▷ Reassure and calm athlete.
▷ Ask athlete if she wants to be helped to sideline.
▷ Wait until athlete can sit up and is ready to move.
▷ Support injured elbow with two hands.
▷ Help athlete slowly stand.
▷ Support athlete and walk slowly to sideline.
▷ Observe athlete's general attitude.
▷ Ask athlete how she feels.

Begin Sideline Evaluation and Care

ELBOW INJURY

ELBOW INJURY

3 Athlete on Sideline

Stop athlete from returning to game.
Remove athletic gear, starting with uninjured arm.

4 Recheck for These Signs & Symptoms

Severe pain

Deformity

Compound fracture or puncture wound

Grating bones

Any Found

Numb hand

No pulse at wrist

None Found

Weak hand

Severe localized tenderness

Painful range of motion

5 Check for These Signs & Symptoms

Swelling

Any Found

Localized tenderness

Limited range of motion

None Found

96

Athlete Needs Emergency Care

▷ Call 911 or transport athlete to medical facility.

▷ Cover all wounds.

▷ Splint elbow.

▷ Don't give food or water.

Athlete Should See a Doctor Today

▷ Follow PRICE Guidelines: protect, rest, ice, compress, elevate.

▷ If necessary, assist athlete home after game.

▷ Report injury to parents or guardian.

▷ Stress potential seriousness of elbow injuries.

▷ Encourage them to take athlete to a doctor today.

▷ Inform them athlete cannot return to play without written medical consent.

Athlete Can Return to Play

▷ If reevaluation is normal after athlete sits for 5 to 10 minutes

▷ If athlete has full, pain-free range of motion

▷ If athlete has normal strength

▷ If athlete performs push-ups without pain

▷ If athlete wants to return to play

Forearm Injury

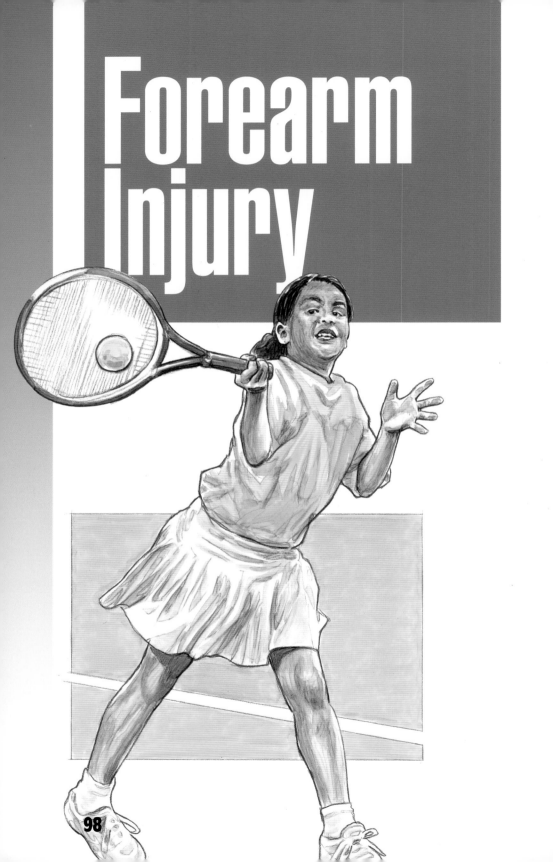

Wrist and forearm fractures, usually caused by an impact to the hand as an athlete tries to break a fall, are the most common extremity injuries you will encounter. An arm that appears deformed should be splinted and the athlete sent for immediate medical evaluation. Nerves run close to the bone; therefore, never try to straighten the arm prior to splinting. More commonly, the injury may not appear severe. Maintain a high index of suspicion and carefully evaluate the athlete. Wrist pain or localized tenderness should be considered a fracture until X-rayed. In most cases, you can splint the arm or wrist and transport the injured athlete to a medical facility yourself.

Possible Injuries

Fractured or dislocated wrist

Fractured forearm
(radius or ulna)

Dr. Steele's Quick Tips

- When treating a severe forearm or wrist injury, splint the arm or wrist where it lies. Do not attempt to straighten any deformity.

- You can assume a forearm or wrist injury has occurred if
  - there is severe localized tenderness over the bone,
  - the athlete has a weak grip,
  - the athlete cannot painlessly twist her arm to turn the palm up or down, or
  - the athlete cannot painlessly bend her wrist completely forward and back.

1 Athlete Down

Don't let athlete move.
Don't move athlete.
Don't bend or turn arm or wrist.
Calm athlete.

2 Check for These Signs & Symptoms

Severe pain
Deformity
Compound fracture or puncture wound
Grating bones
Numb hand
No pulse at wrist
Weak hand
Severe localized tenderness
Painful range of motion

Any Found

None Found

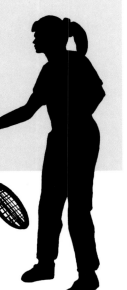

Athlete Needs Emergency Care

▷ Call 911 or transport athlete to medical facility.
▷ Don't try to straighten a deformity.
▷ Cover all wounds.
▷ Splint arm and wrist.
▷ Don't give food or water.

Assist Athlete to Sideline

▷ Reassure and calm athlete.
▷ Ask athlete if she wants to be helped to sideline.
▷ Wait until athlete can sit up and is ready to move.
▷ Support injured forearm or wrist with both hands.
▷ Help athlete slowly stand.
▷ Support athlete and walk slowly to sideline.
▷ Observe athlete's general attitude.
▷ Ask athlete how she feels.

Begin Sideline Evaluation and Care ▶

FOREARM INJURY

FOREARM INJURY

3 Athlete on Sideline

Stop athlete from returning to game.

Remove athletic gear, starting with uninjured arm.

4 Recheck for These Signs & Symptoms

Severe pain

Deformity

Compound fracture or puncture wound

Grating bones

Any Found

Numb hand

No pulse at wrist

None Found

Weak hand

Severe localized tenderness

Painful range of motion

5 Check for These Signs & Symptoms

Swelling

Any Found

Localized tenderness

Limited range of motion

None Found

Athlete Needs Emergency Care

▷ Call 911 or transport athlete to medical facility.
▷ Cover all wounds.
▷ Splint arm and wrist.
▷ Don't give food or water.

Athlete Should See a Doctor Today

▷ Follow PRICE Guidelines: protect, rest, ice, compress, elevate.
▷ If necessary, assist athlete home after game.
▷ Report injury to parents or guardian.
▷ Stress potential seriousness of forearm injuries.
▷ Encourage them to take athlete to a doctor today.
▷ Inform them athlete cannot return to play without written medical consent.

Athlete Can Return to Play

▷ If reevaluation is normal after athlete sits for 5 to 10 minutes
▷ If athlete has full, pain-free range of motion
▷ If athlete has normal strength
▷ If athlete performs push-ups without pain
▷ If athlete wants to return to play

FOREARM INJURY

103

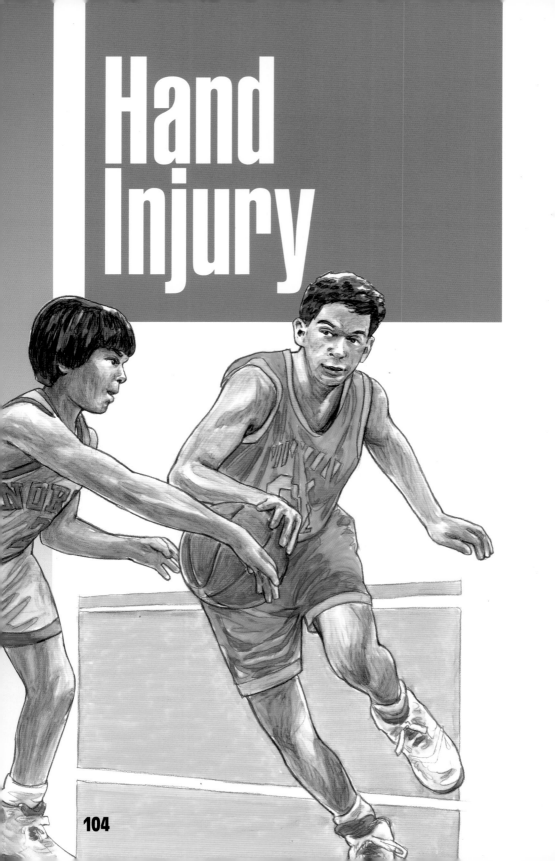

Hand Injury

njuries to the hand may result in fractures of the bone, dislocations of the small joints, or a combination of both. Two arteries and two nerves run along each side of the bones in the fingers. It is unwise to try to straighten a deformed finger or thumb because you may cause further damage. It is better to splint the finger in its abnormal position.

Possible Injuries

Fractured or dislocated finger or thumb

Broken bone in hand

Torn ligaments

What appear to be small cuts near a deformed finger may actually be where the bone has punctured the skin. To keep the bone from becoming contaminated, cover the cuts with sterile sponges immediately. Less severe but potentially serious fractures may be more difficult to detect if there is no deformity. Carefully examine the injured finger for localized tenderness and loss of motion. You can splint the finger or thumb and transport the athlete to a medical facility yourself for almost all hand injuries.

Dr. Steele's Quick Tips

■ When treating finger or thumb injuries, splint the finger or thumb as it lies. Do not attempt to straighten any deformity.

■ You can assume a finger or thumb injury has occurred if

   ■ the athlete cannot fully straighten and bend his fingers without pain, or

   ■ there is localized tenderness along the bone.

1 Athlete Down

▷▷▷ Don't let athlete move.
Don't move athlete.
Don't straighten or bend fingers or thumb.
Calm athlete.

2 Check for These Signs & Symptoms

▷▷▷ Severe pain
Deformity
Compound fracture or puncture wound
Grating bones
Numb finger or thumb
Severe localized tenderness
Painful range of motion

Any Found ▷

None Found ▷

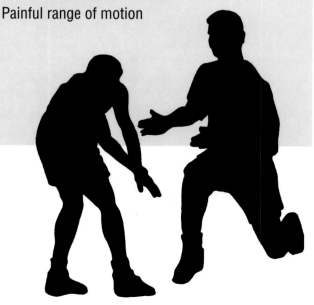

Athlete Needs Emergency Care

▷▷ Transport athlete to medical facility.
▷▷ Don't try to straighten a deformity.
▷▷ Cover all wounds.
▷▷ Splint finger or thumb.
▷▷ Don't give food or water.

 ## Assist Athlete to Sideline

▷▷ Reassure and calm athlete.
▷▷ Ask athlete if he wants to be helped to sideline.
▷▷ Wait until athlete can sit up and is ready to move.
▷▷ Support injured hand.
▷▷ Help athlete slowly stand.
▷▷ Support athlete and walk slowly to sideline.
▷▷ Observe athlete's general attitude.
▷▷ Ask athlete how he feels.

Begin Sideline Evaluation and Care ▶

HAND INJURY

3 Athlete on Sideline

▷▷ Stop athlete from returning to game.

▷▷ Remove athletic gear, starting with uninjured arm.

4 Recheck for These Signs & Symptoms

▷▷ Severe pain

▷▷ Deformity

▷▷ Compound fracture or puncture wound

▷▷ Grating bones

▷▷ Numb finger or thumb

▷▷ Severe localized tenderness

▷▷ Painful range of motion

Any Found ▷

None Found ▷

5 Check for These Signs & Symptoms

▷▷ Swelling

▷▷ Localized tenderness

▷▷ Limited range of motion

Any Found ▷

None Found ▷

Athlete Needs Emergency Care

Transport athlete to medical facility.

Cover all wounds.

Splint finger or thumb.

Don't give food or water.

Athlete Should See a Doctor Today

Follow PRICE Guidelines: protect, rest, ice, compress, elevate.

If necessary, assist athlete home after game.

Report injury to parents or guardian.

Stress potential seriousness of hand injuries.

Encourage them to take athlete to a doctor today.

Inform them athlete cannot return to play without written medical consent.

Athlete Can Return to Play

If reevaluation is normal after athlete sits for 5 to 10 minutes

If athlete has full, pain-free range of motion

If athlete has normal strength

If athlete wants to return to play

HAND INJURY

Hip Injury

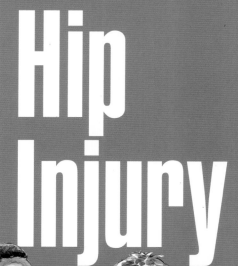
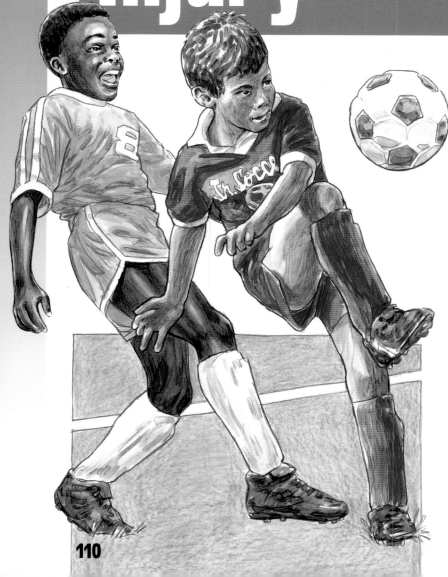

F
ractures to the hip, fe-
mur, and pelvis are the
most serious of the ex-
tremity injuries. Significant
internal bleeding may oc-
cur, requiring immediate
medical attention. In most
cases, the athlete will not be
able to move. Do not attempt
to straighten a deformity;
major arteries and nerves run adjacent to the bone and you could
cause further injury. The hip growth plate of children ages 10 to
16 may fracture without a fall. Any athlete in this age group who
complains of hip or knee pain and who limps while running
should be evaluated for this subtle injury by a medical professional.

Possible Injuries

Fractured or dislocated hip

Fracture above the knee

Fractured pelvis

Fractured growth plate

Dr. Steele's Quick Tips

■ When treating a severe hip injury, do not move the athlete,
  attempt to straighten a deformity, or splint the leg. Immobilize the hip and leg and wait for emergency help.

■ For a less serious injury, check for painful or limited
  motion by asking the athlete to
  - ■ bend his knee to his chest,
  - ■ turn his foot in and out completely, and
  - ■ lift his leg while lying on the ground.

■ A young athlete with knee or hip pain who limps while
  running may have sustained a fracture to the hip growth
  plate. He should receive professional medical attention
  immediately.

HIP INJURY

1 Athlete Down

▷▷▷ Don't let athlete move.

Don't move athlete.

Don't straighten or turn leg or hip.

Calm athlete.

2 Check for These Signs & Symptoms

▷ Severe pain

▷ Deformity

▷ Compound fracture or puncture wound

▷ Grating bones

▷ Numb foot

▷ No pulse at ankle

▷ Weak leg

▷ Severe localized tenderness

▷ Painful range of motion

Any Found ▷

None Found ▷

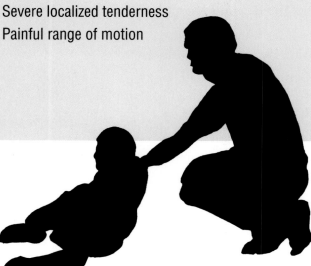

Athlete Needs Emergency Care

Call 911.
Don't try to straighten a deformity.
Cover all wounds.
Protect and stabilize hip and leg.
Don't move athlete.
Don't give food or water.

Assist Athlete to Sideline

Reassure and calm athlete.
Ask athlete if he wants to be helped to sideline.
Wait until athlete can sit up and is ready to move.
Help athlete slowly stand.
If pain exists, have athlete avoid bearing weight.
Support athlete and walk slowly to sideline.
Observe athlete's balance and general attitude.
Ask athlete how he feels.

Begin Sideline Evaluation and Care ▶

HIP INJURY

3 Athlete on Sideline

▷ Stop athlete from returning to game.
▷ Remove athletic gear, starting with uninjured leg.

4 Recheck for These Signs & Symptoms

▷ Severe pain
▷ Deformity
▷ Compound fracture or puncture wound
▷ Grating bones
▷ Numb foot
▷ No pulse at ankle
▷ Weak leg
▷ Severe localized tenderness
▷ Painful range of motion

Any Found ▷

None Found ▷

5 Check for These Signs & Symptoms

▷ Swelling
▷ Limping
▷ Localized tenderness
▷ Limited range of motion

Any Found ▷

None Found ▷

Athlete Needs Emergency Care

▷ Call 911 or transport athlete to medical facility.

▷ Cover all wounds.

▷ Protect and stabilize hip and leg.

▷ Don't give food or water.

 ## Athlete Should See a Doctor Today

▷ Follow PRICE Guidelines: protect, rest, ice, compress, elevate.

▷ If necessary, assist athlete home after game.

▷ Report injury to parents or guardian.

▷ Stress potential seriousness of hip injuries.

▷ Encourage them to take athlete to a doctor today.

▷ Inform them athlete cannot return to play without written medical consent.

 ## Athlete Can Return to Play

▷ If reevaluation is normal after athlete sits for 5 to 10 minutes

▷ If athlete has full, pain-free range of motion

▷ If athlete has normal strength

▷ If athlete performs one-leg hops, jumping jacks, crossovers, and figure eights without pain

▷ If athlete sprints without limping

▷ If athlete wants to return to play

HIP INJURY

115

Knee Injury

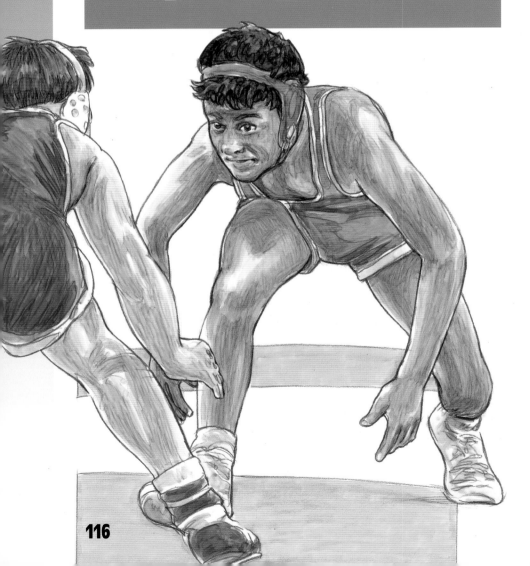

Knee injuries can be very serious. Because a major nerve and a major artery run close to the bone, a deformed or extremely painful knee signals a potentially dangerous injury. In this case, do not move the athlete or his knee. Call for emergency help and wait for professionals to move and transport the athlete to the hospital.

Possible Injuries

Dislocated knee

Fracture above or below the knee

Dislocated kneecap

Torn ligament

Bruised knee

Fortunately, most knee injuries are not this serious. Ligament injuries—usually accompanied by an audible *pop*—are frequently the result of a simple twisted knee. Although he may be able to walk comfortably and may even ask to return to competition, an athlete with potential ligament damage should not return to action without first being evaluated by a medical professional. You may decide to transport an athlete with a less serious knee injury to a medical facility yourself.

Dr. Steele's Quick Tips

- When treating a severe knee injury, don't move the athlete, attempt to straighten a deformity, or splint the knee. Immobilize the knee and wait for emergency help.

- You can assume ligament damage has occurred if
  - the athlete felt or heard a *pop* in the knee joint,
  - the athlete's knee buckles or feels unstable under normal loads, or
  - the athlete's knee swells.

- Check for painful or limited motion by asking the athlete to bend and straighten his knee completely.

KNEE INJURY

1 Athlete Down

▷▷▷ Don't let athlete move.
Don't move athlete.
Don't straighten or bend knee.
Calm athlete.

2 Check for These Signs & Symptoms

▷▷▷▷▷▷▷▷▷ Severe pain
Deformity
Compound fracture or puncture wound
Grating bones
Numb foot
No pulse at ankle
Weak foot or ankle
Severe localized tenderness
Painful range of motion

Any Found ▷

None Found ▷

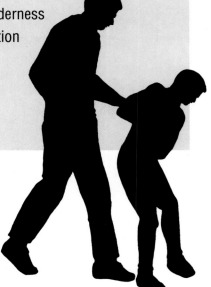

Athlete Needs Emergency Care

▷ Call 911 or transport athlete to medical facility.
▷ Don't try to straighten a deformity.
▷ Cover all wounds.
▷ Protect and stabilize knee.
▷ Don't move athlete.
▷ Don't give food or water.

Assist Athlete to Sideline

▷ Reassure and calm athlete.
▷ Ask athlete if he wants to be helped to sideline.
▷ Wait until athlete can sit up and is ready to move.
▷ Help athlete slowly stand.
▷ If pain exists, have athlete avoid bearing weight.
▷ Support athlete and walk slowly to sideline.
▷ Observe athlete's balance and general attitude.
▷ Ask athlete how he feels.

Begin Sideline Evaluation and Care ▶

KNEE INJURY

KNEE INJURY

3 Athlete on Sideline

▷ Stop athlete from returning to game.
▷ Remove athletic gear, starting with uninjured leg.

4 Recheck for These Signs & Symptoms

▷ Severe pain
▷ Deformity
▷ Compound fracture or puncture wound
▷ Grating bones
▷ Numb foot
▷ No pulse at ankle
▷ Weak foot or ankle
▷ Severe localized tenderness
▷ Painful range of motion

Any Found ▷

None Found ▷

5 Check for These Signs & Symptoms

▷ Swelling
▷ Limping
▷ Localized tenderness
▷ Unstable knee
▷ Limited range of motion
▷ Athlete felt or heard a *pop*

Any Found ▷

None Found ▷

Athlete Needs Emergency Care

▷ Call 911 or transport athlete to medical facility.

▷ Cover all wounds.

▷ Splint knee.

▷ Don't give food or water.

Athlete Should See a Doctor Today

▷ Follow PRICE Guidelines: protect, rest, ice, compress, elevate.

▷ If necessary, assist athlete home after game.

▷ Report injury to parents or guardian.

▷ Stress potential seriousness of knee injuries.

▷ Encourage them to take athlete to a doctor today.

▷ Inform them athlete cannot return to play without written medical consent.

Athlete Can Return to Play

▷ If reevaluation is normal after athlete sits for 5 to 10 minutes

▷ If athlete has full, pain-free range of motion

▷ If athlete has normal strength

▷ If athlete performs one-leg hops, jumping jacks, crossovers, and figure eights without pain

▷ If athlete sprints without limping

▷ If athlete wants to return to play

KNEE INJURY

Lower Leg Injury

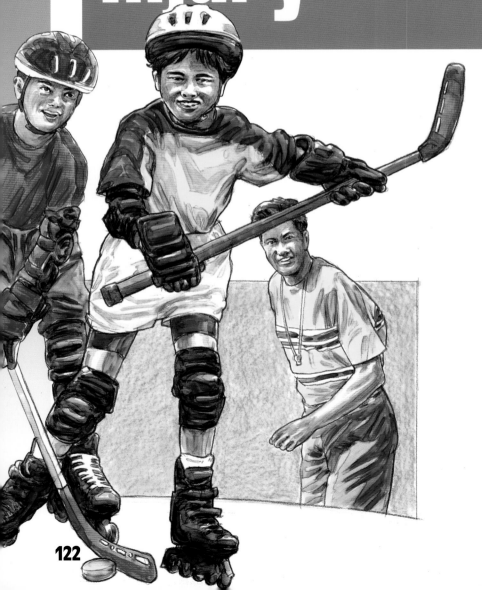

A twist or blow to the lower leg may result in a fracture of the tibia (large bone), fibula (small bone), or both. Because the bones are very close to the skin, the sharp edge of the broken bone often pierces the skin and may damage the arteries and nerves that run adjacent to the bone. Therefore, consider all cuts in the area of a suspected fracture to be open wounds linking directly to the fracture. Cover the wound immediately to prevent contamination. In the case of a deformed leg, splint the leg where it lies and do not attempt to straighten it.

Occasionally, when only the fibula fractures, the athlete may still be able to walk or run. Carefully examine the outside of the leg for localized tenderness and watch for limping so you won't miss this serious injury. You may decide to transport athletes with less serious leg injuries to a medical facility yourself.

Possible Injuries

Fractured lower leg
(tibia or fibula)

Bruised leg

Dr. Steele's Quick Tips

■ When treating severe lower leg injuries, check carefully for puncture wounds, then splint the leg where it lies. Do not attempt to straighten any deformity or move the athlete to the sideline.

■ You can assume a leg injury has occurred if
   ■ the athlete exhibits severe localized tenderness, or
   ■ the athlete limps while running.

1 Athlete Down

▷▷▷ Don't let athlete move.
Don't move athlete.
Don't straighten or bend leg.
Calm athlete.

2 Check for These Signs & Symptoms

▷▷▷
▷▷▷▷▷▷
Severe pain
Deformity
Compound fracture or puncture wound
Grating bones
Numb foot
No pulse at ankle
Weak foot
Severe localized tenderness
Painful range of motion

Any Found ▷

None Found ▷

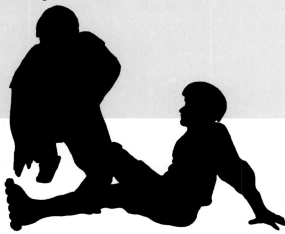

Athlete Needs Emergency Care

▷ Call 911 or transport athlete to medical facility.
▷ Cover all wounds.
▷ Splint leg.
▷ Don't move athlete.
▷ Don't give food or water.

Assist Athlete to Sideline

▷ Reassure and calm athlete.
▷ Ask athlete if he wants to be helped to sideline.
▷ Wait until athlete can sit up and is ready to move.
▷ Help athlete slowly stand.
▷ If pain exists, have athlete avoid bearing weight.
▷ Support athlete and walk slowly to sideline.
▷ Observe athlete's balance and general attitude.
▷ Ask athlete how he feels.

Begin Sideline Evaluation and Care

LOWER LEG INJURY

3 Athlete on Sideline

▷ Stop athlete from returning to game.
Remove athletic gear, starting with uninjured leg.

4 Recheck for These Signs & Symptoms

▷ Severe pain
▷ Deformity
▷ Compound fracture or puncture wound
▷ Grating bones
▷ Numb foot
▷ No pulse at ankle
▷ Weak foot
▷ Severe localized tenderness
▷ Painful range of motion

Any Found ▷

None Found ▷

5 Check for These Signs & Symptoms

▷ Swelling
▷ Limping
▷ Localized tenderness
▷ Limited range of motion

Any Found ▷

None Found ▷

Athlete Needs Emergency Care

▷ Call 911 or transport athlete to medical facility.

▷ Cover all wounds.

▷ Splint leg.

▷ Don't give food or water.

 ## Athlete Should See a Doctor Today

▷ Follow PRICE Guidelines: protect, rest, ice, compress, elevate.

▷ If necessary, assist athlete home after game.

▷ Report injury to parents or guardian.

▷ Stress potential seriousness of lower leg injuries.

▷ Encourage them to take athlete to a doctor today.

▷ Inform them athlete cannot return to play without written medical consent.

 ## Athlete Can Return to Play

▷ If reevaluation is normal after athlete sits for 5 to 10 minutes

▷ If athlete has full, pain-free range of motion

▷ If athlete has normal strength

▷ If athlete performs one-leg hops, jumping jacks, crossovers, and figure eights without pain

▷ If athlete sprints without limping

▷ If athlete wants to return to play

LOWER LEG INJURY

Ankle Injury

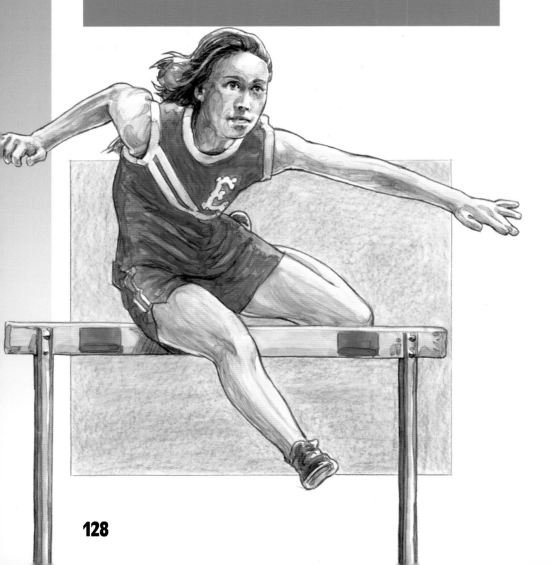

Bones around the ankle may be fractured when the ankle is twisted. Without the stability of the bones, the ankle may go out of joint, which creates a serious deformity. Arteries and nerves that run close to the bones can be torn or stretched if the ankle is dislocated, and sharp edges of bone can tear the skin. Cover all cuts immediately to prevent contamination of the bone. Do not attempt to straighten the deformity, because you may cause further damage to arteries and nerves. Wait on the field for emergency help.

Possible Injuries

Fractured or dislocated ankle

Torn ligament

Most ankle injuries are not that serious. However, if the athlete heard a *pop* or *crack* or has pain with movement, pain with weight bearing, or swelling, she probably has a ligament tear or a fracture. She should be promptly evaluated by trained medical personnel. You may decide to transport athletes with less serious ankle injuries to a medical facility yourself.

Dr. Steele's Quick Tips

■ When treating severe ankle injuries, check carefully for puncture wounds, then splint the ankle where it lies. Do not attempt to straighten any deformity or move the athlete to the sideline.

■ Check for painful or limited motion by asking the athlete to
   ■ move her ankle up and down and
   ■ rotate her ankle from side to side.

ANKLE INJURY

1 Athlete Down

▷▷▷▷ Don't let athlete move.
Don't move athlete.
Don't bend or twist ankle.
Calm athlete.

2 Check for These Signs & Symptoms

▷▷▷▷▷▷▷▷▷ Severe pain
Deformity
Compound fracture or puncture wound
Grating bones
Numb foot
No pulse at ankle
Weak toes
Severe localized tenderness
Painful range of motion

Any Found ▷

None Found ▷

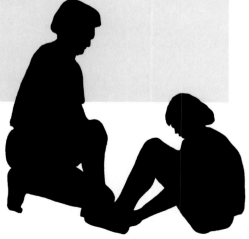

Athlete Needs Emergency Care

▷ Call 911 or transport athlete to medical facility.
▷ Cover all wounds.
▷ Splint ankle.
▷ Don't move athlete.
▷ Don't give food or water.

Assist Athlete to Sideline

▷ Reassure and calm athlete.
▷ Ask athlete if she wants to be helped to sideline.
▷ Wait until athlete can sit up and is ready to move.
▷ Help athlete slowly stand.
▷ If pain exists, have athlete avoid bearing weight.
▷ Support athlete and walk slowly to sideline.
▷ Observe athlete's balance and general attitude.
▷ Ask athlete how she feels.

Begin Sideline Evaluation and Care ▶

3 Athlete on Sideline

Stop athlete from returning to game.

Remove shoe and sock carefully.

Remove athletic gear, starting with uninjured leg.

4 Recheck for These Signs & Symptoms

Severe pain

Deformity

Compound fracture or puncture wound

Grating bones

Any Found

Numb foot

No pulse at ankle

None Found

Weak toes

Severe localized tenderness

Painful range of motion

5 Check for These Signs & Symptoms

Swelling

Limping

Any Found

Localized tenderness

Limited range of motion

None Found

Athlete felt or heard a *pop* or *crack*

ANKLE INJURY

Athlete Needs Emergency Care

▷ Call 911 or transport athlete to medical facility.

▷ Cover all wounds.

▷ Splint ankle.

▷ Don't give food or water.

Athlete Should See a Doctor Today

▷ Follow PRICE Guidelines: protect, rest, ice, compress, elevate.

▷ If necessary, assist athlete home after game.

▷ Report injury to parents or guardian.

▷ Stress potential seriousness of ankle injuries.

▷ Encourage them to take athlete to a doctor today.

▷ Inform them athlete cannot return to play without written medical consent.

Athlete Can Return to Play

▷ If reevaluation is normal after athlete sits for 5 to 10 minutes

▷ If athlete has full, pain-free range of motion

▷ If athlete has normal strength

▷ If athlete performs one-leg hops, jumping jacks, crossovers, and figure eights without pain

▷ If athlete sprints without limping

▷ If athlete wants to return to play

133

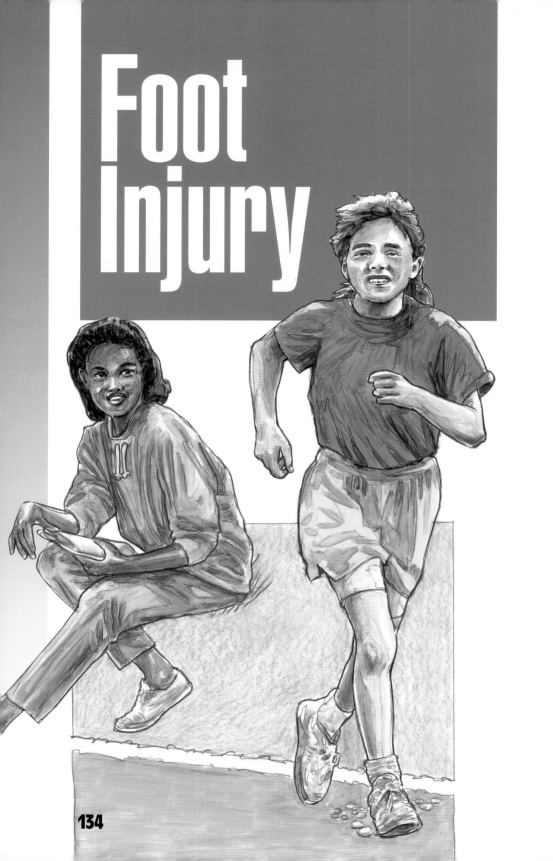

Foot Injury

Severe foot injuries are uncommon in sport. Most foot fractures occur with a twist of the ankle or foot or because of a direct blow to the foot. Occasionally, a fractured bone in the foot or toe will penetrate the skin. Immediately cover the wound to prevent contamination of the bone. In the case of deformed toes, do not attempt to straighten them, but splint them as they are.

Possible Injuries

Fractured or dislocated toe

Fractured bone in foot

Torn ligament

In most cases, you can splint the foot and transport the athlete to a medical facility yourself.

Dr. Steele's Quick Tips

■ When treating severe foot injuries, check carefully for puncture wounds, then splint the foot or toe where it lies. Do not attempt to straighten any deformity.

■ You can assume a foot injury has occurred if

■ the athlete felt or heard a *pop* or *crack,*
■ the athlete cannot bear weight without pain, or
■ the athlete has tenderness over the bone.

■ A twisted ankle can cause a fracture in the side of the foot, and the injury is often mistaken for an ankle sprain. Examine the side of the foot for localized tenderness to check for a fracture in this area.

FOOT INJURY

1 Athlete Down

▸▸▸ Don't let athlete move.
Don't move athlete.
Don't straighten or bend foot.
Calm athlete.

2 Check for These Signs & Symptoms

▸▸▸ Severe pain
Deformity
Compound fracture or puncture wound
Grating bones
Numb toes
No pulse at ankle
Severe localized tenderness
Painful range of motion

Any Found ▸

None Found ▸

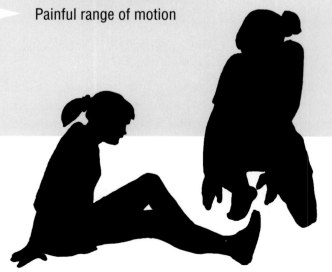

Athlete Needs Emergency Care

▷ Transport athlete to medical facility.
▷ Cover all wounds.
▷ Splint foot or toe.
▷ Don't give food or water.

 ## Assist Athlete to Sideline

▷ Reassure and calm athlete.
▷ Ask athlete if she wants to be helped to sideline.
▷ Wait until athlete can sit up and is ready to move.
▷ Help athlete slowly stand.
▷ If pain exists, have athlete avoid bearing weight.
▷ Support athlete and walk slowly to sideline.
▷ Observe athlete's balance and general attitude.
▷ Ask athlete how she feels.

Begin Sideline Evaluation and Care ▶

FOOT INJURY

FOOT INJURY

3 Athlete on Sideline

▷▷▷ Stop athlete from returning to game.

Remove shoe and sock carefully.

Remove athletic gear, starting with uninjured leg.

4 Recheck for These Signs & Symptoms

▷▷ Severe pain

Deformity

Compound fracture or puncture wound

Grating bones

Numb toes

No pulse at ankle

Severe localized tenderness

Painful range of motion

Any Found

None Found

5 Check for These Signs & Symptoms

▷▷ Swelling

Limping

Localized tenderness

Limited range of motion

Athlete felt or heard a *pop* or *crack*

Any Found

None Found

Athlete Needs Emergency Care

Transport athlete to medical facility.

Cover all wounds.

Splint foot or toe.

Don't give food or water.

Athlete Should See a Doctor Today

Follow PRICE Guidelines: protect, rest, ice, compress, elevate.

If necessary, assist athlete home after game.

Report injury to parents or guardian.

Stress potential seriousness of foot injuries.

Encourage them to take athlete to a doctor today.

Inform them athlete cannot return to play without written medical consent.

Athlete Can Return to Play

If reevaluation is normal after athlete sits for 5 to 10 minutes

If athlete has full, pain-free range of motion

If athlete has normal strength

If athlete performs one-leg hops, jumping jacks, crossovers, and figure eights without pain

If athlete sprints without limping

If athlete wants to return to play

FOOT INJURY

INJURY PREVENTION AND CARE RESOURCES

You can contact the following organizations for information about sports injuries and injury prevention, as well as CPR and first aid courses in your area.

American Academy of Family Physicians (AAFP)
8880 Ward Parkway
Kansas City, MO 64114
(816) 333-9700
(800) 274-2237

American Academy of Orthopaedic Surgeons (AAOS)
6300 North River Road
Rosemont, IL 60018-4226
(708) 823-7186

American Academy of Pediatrics (AAP)
141 Northwest Point Boulevard
Box 927
Elk Grove Village, IL 60009-0927
(800) 433-9016 (outside Illinois)
(800) 421-0589 (within Illinois)

American Athletic Trainers Association (AATA)
660 West Duarte Road
Arcadia, CA 91007
(818) 445-1978

American College of Sports Medicine (ACSM)
Box 1440
Indianapolis, IN 46206-1440
(317) 637-9200

American Heart Association
7272 Greenville Avenue
Dallas, TX 75231-4596
(214) 373-6300

American Medical Society for Sports Medicine (AMSSM)
7611 Elmwood Avenue, Suite 201
Middleton, WI 53562
(608) 831-4484

American Orthopaedic Society for Sports Medicine (AOSSM)
6300 North River Road, Suite 300
Rosemont, IL 60018-4263
(708) 318-7330

American Red Cross
431 18th Street NW
Washington, DC 20006
(202) 737-8300

National Athletic Trainers' Association Inc. (NATA)
2952 Stemmons Freeway, Suite 200
Dallas, TX 75247-6103
(214) 637-6282

National Youth Sports Foundation for the Prevention of Athletic Injuries Inc. (NYSFPAI)
10 Meredith Circle
Needham, MA 02192-1946
(617) 449-2499

Young Men's Christian Association
101 N. Wacker Drive
Chicago, IL 60606
(312) 977-0031
(800) 872-9622

ABOUT THE AUTHOR

Marshall K. Steele III, MD, has been caring for high school, college, and young athletes since 1977. In 1983 he started the first comprehensive program in Maryland for athletic trainers working with high school and youth sports. Under the program, each high school in Anne Arundel County was assigned an athletic trainer who visited the school at least twice weekly. Dr. Steele also recruited volunteer team physicians throughout the county for high school football games.

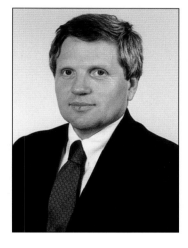

Dr. Steele has presented many lectures to coaches and primary care physicians and received several awards, including the Robert Pascal Service Award for special service to high school athletes and the Anne Arundel County Coaches Award. A member of the American Academy of Orthopaedic Surgeons and the American College of Sports Medicine (ACSM), he has been a member of the ACSM's Committee on Youth Clinics, a state commissioner on the Maryland Physical Fitness Commission, and a national advisory board member for Caremark, Inc. He also was a sports medicine physician at the 1984 Olympic Games.

Dr. Steele holds a medical degree from the University of Maryland and is president of the Orthopaedic and Sports Medicine Center in Annapolis, MD.

Related Books From Human Kinetics

Coaching Youth Sports Series

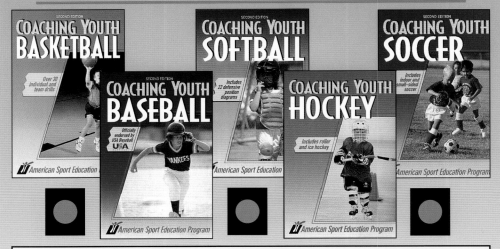

COACHING YOUTH BASKETBALL
SECOND EDITION
Over 30 individual and team drills
American Sport Education Program

COACHING YOUTH SOFTBALL
SECOND EDITION
Includes 22 defensive position diagrams
American Sport Education

COACHING YOUTH SOCCER
SECOND EDITION
Includes indoor and small-sided soccer
American Sport Education Program

COACHING YOUTH BASEBALL
SECOND EDITION
Officially endorsed by USA Baseball
American Sport Education Program

COACHING YOUTH HOCKEY
Includes roller and ice hockey
American Sport Education Program

Forthcoming Titles in the Coaching Youth Sports Series:

Volleyball	Skiing	Football	Gymnastics
Swimming	Wrestling	Tennis	

✚ Sport First Aid

An excellent companion to *Sideline Help*, *Sport First Aid* features explicit, step-by-step first aid procedures for nearly 100 athletic injuries, highlighted by more than 250 illustrations. Of special interest is a chapter devoted to the 39 musculoskeletal injuries most frequently suffered by athletes.

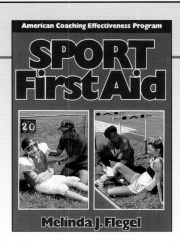

American Coaching Effectiveness Program

SPORT First Aid

Melinda J. Flegel

To request more information or to place your order, U.S. customers call **TOLL-FREE 1-800-747-4457**.

Customers outside the U.S. use appropriate telephone number/address shown in the front of this book.

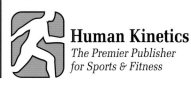

Human Kinetics
The Premier Publisher for Sports & Fitness